Researching Families and Communities

Recent years have seen a concern with how family and community relationships have changed across the generations, whether for better or worse, and particularly how they have been affected by social and economic developments. But how can we think about and research the nature of the present in relation to the past and vice versa?

Researching Families and Communities: Social and generational change explores the concepts and perspectives that guide research and the methods used to explore change during the latter half of the twentieth century and into the new millennium. It highlights the complexities of continuities alongside change, the importance of the perspectives that shape investigation, and the need to engage with situated data. This edited text includes contributions from experts in their field who:

- address these overarching trends;
- explore the possibilities and practices of secondary analysis or replication studies, as well as longitudinal large-scale data sets;
- discuss varied aspects of family and community life, including sexuality, ethnicity, parenting resources, older people, intergenerational family life, solo living, and many others.

This book will appeal to academics and students interested in family and community across a range of social science disciplines, and to those in the social research field.

Rosalind Edwards is Professor in Social Policy and Director of the Families & Social Capital Research Group at London South Bank University. She has researched and published widely in the field of family studies.

Relationships & Resources
Series Editors: Janet Holland and Rosalind Edwards
London South Bank University

A key contemporary political and intellectual issue is the link between the relationships that people have and the resources to which they have access. When people share a sense of identity, hold similar values, trust each other, and reciprocally do things for each other, this has an impact on the social, political, and economic cohesion of the society in which they live. So, are changes in contemporary society leading to deterioration in the link between relationships and resources, new and innovative forms of linking, or merely the reproduction of enduring inequalities? Consideration of relationships and resources raises key theoretical and empirical issues around change and continuity over time as well as time use, the consequences of globalisation and individualisation for intimate and broader social relations, and location and space in terms of communities and neighbourhoods. The books in this series are concerned with elaborating these issues and will form a body of work that will contribute to academic and political debate.

Other titles include:

Marginalised Mothers
Exploring Working Class Experiences of Parenting
Val Gillies

Moving On
Bren Neale and Jennifer Flowerdew

Sibling Identity and Relationships
Sisters and Brothers
Rosalind Edwards, Lucy Hadfield, Helen Laucey, and Melanie Mauthner

Teenagers' Citizenship
Experiences and Education
Susie Weller

Researching Families and Communities

Social and generational change

Edited by Rosalind Edwards

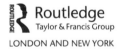

Routledge
Taylor & Francis Group

LONDON AND NEW YORK

First published 2008
by Routledge
2 Park Square, Milton Park, Abingdon, Oxon OX14 4RN

Simultaneously published in the USA and Canada
by Routledge
270 Madison Ave, New York, NY 10016

Routledge is an imprint of the Taylor & Francis Group, an informa business

Typeset in Sabon by
GreenGate Publishing Services, Tonbridge, Kent
Printed and bound in Great Britain by
TJ International Ltd, Padstow, Cornwall

British Library Cataloguing in Publication Data
A catalogue record for this book is available from the British Library

Library of Congress Cataloging-in-Publication Data
Researching families and communities : social and generational change / [edited by] Rosalind Edwards.
    p. cm. — (Relationships and resources)
    ISBN 978-0-415-42711-1 — ISBN 978-0-415-42712-8 1. Family. 2. Community-based family services.
3. Social change. 4. Generations. I. Edwards, Rosalind.
    HQ518.R434 2008
    307.09'04501—dc22   *2007043300*

ISBN 10: 0-415-42711-8 (hbk)
ISBN 10: 0-415-42712-6 (pbk)
ISBN 10: 0-203-92811-3 (ebk)
ISBN 13: 978-0-415-42711-1 (hbk)
ISBN 13: 978-0-415-42712-8 (pbk)
ISBN 13: 978-0-203-92811-3 (ebk)

Contents

Contributors

Joanna Bornat is Professor of Oral History in the Faculty of Health and Social Care at the Open University. Over the years she has researched and published in the area of remembering in late life. She has edited or jointly edited *Reminiscence Reviewed* (Open University Press, 1994), *Oral History, Health and Welfare* (Routledge, 2000), *The Turn to Biographical Methods in Social Science* (Routledge, 2000), and *Biographical Methods and Professional Practice*. She is currently researching the contribution of overseas-trained South Asian doctors to the geriatric speciality and is participating with a project on the oldest generation in 'Timescapes', a consortium of researchers interested in the secondary analysis of longitudinal research.

Joan Chandler is Professor of Sociology at the University of Plymouth. She has a sustained interest in families and households that led to her engagement in research projects on living alone. She has also published recently in the area of children and consumption.

Nickie Charles is Professor and Director of the Centre for the Study of Women and Gender in the Sociology Department at the University of Warwick. She and her co-authors are writing a book entitled *Families in Transition: 'The Family and Social Change' Revisited*, which is based on their re-study of a classic piece of research on families carried out in Swansea in the early 1960s. The re-study was funded by the ESRC (R000238454) and the book is due to be published in 2008 by Policy Press. She is currently working with colleagues at Swansea University, researching gender and political processes in the context of devolution. Her most recent book is *Gender in Modern Britain* (Oxford University Press, 2002). Other books include *Feminism, the State and Social Policy* (Macmillan, 2000), *Gender Divisions and Social Change* (Harvester Wheatsheaf, 1993), and *Women, Food and Families* (Manchester University Press, 1988).

Graham Crow is Professor of Sociology at the University of Southampton, where he is Deputy Director of the ESRC National Centre for Research Methods. He is also co-editor of the journal *Sociology*. His research interests include the sociology of families and communities, comparative sociology, sociological theory, and research methods. His most recent book is *The Art of Sociological Argument* (Palgrave, 2005).

Charlotte Aull Davies is Senior Lecturer in the Department of Sociology and Anthropology at the University of Swansea. She has researched and published on nationalism and national identity, learning disabilities and personal identity, understandings of personhood and community care policies, feminism and nationalism, the Welsh language and identity, and performance and ritual in the Welsh National Eisteddfod. She is currently involved in a major project looking at gender and political processes in the context of devolution. Her published books include *Welsh Nationalism in the Twentieth Century: The Ethnic Option and the Modern State* (Praeger, 1989), *Reflexive Ethnography* (Routledge, 2008), and *Welsh Communities: New Ethnographic Perspectives* (co-edited with S. Jones, University of Wales Press, 2003).

Brian Dodgeon is a Senior Research Fellow at the Centre for Longitudinal Studies at the Institute of Education, London. He has conducted research using the Longitudinal Study since 1990 and has published widely in a number of areas where the LS has been utilised.

Rosalind Edwards is Professor in Social Policy and Director of the Families & Social Capital Research Group at London South Bank University. She has researched and published widely in the field of family studies. She is currently researching 'mixed' parenting (i.e. race, ethnicity and faith) and children and young people's sibling and friendship relationships over time as part of the five-year 'Timescapes' qualitative longitudinal research consortium. Recent publications include: *Assessing Social Capital* (co-edited with J. Holland and J. Franklin, Cambridge Scholars Press, 2007) and *Sibling Identity and Relationships: Sisters and Brothers* (with L. Hadfield, H. Lucey and M. Mauthner, Routledge, 2006). She is also founding and co-editor of the *International Journal of Social Research Methodology*.

Val Gillies is a Senior Research Fellow in the Families and Social Capital Research Group at London South Bank University. She has researched and published in the areas of family and parenting, producing various journal articles and book chapters on social class, social policy, young people's family lives, family, and social change, as well as qualitative research methods. Her first sole-authored book is *Marginalised Mothers: Exploring Working Class Parenting* (Routledge, 2007). She is currently conducting research with pupils with challenging behaviour.

Harry Goulbourne is Professor of Sociology in the Faculty of Arts and Human Sciences at London South Bank University. He has taught at the universities of Dar-es-Salaam (Tanzania), the West Indies (Jamaica), Warwick, and Gloucestershire. He has also conducted research in Africa, the Caribbean, and Britain. His publications over the last three decades reflect a diversity of interests in sociology and politics, including political theory and development, nationalism, diasporic studies, ethnicity, race and racism, and family studies.

Chris Harris is emeritus professor of Sociology at the University of Swansea. He is co-author of *The Family and Social Change* (RKP, 1965) and author of *Kinship* (Open University Press, 1990), among other publications on the family.

Denise Hawkes is a Research Officer at the Centre for Longitudinal Studies at the Institute of Education, University of London. Her work focuses on the use and application of twin and longitudinal data in understanding the effects of family background and individual characteristics on educational achievement, income, employment, and early motherhood.

Moira Maconachie is a Senior Research Fellow in the School of Law and Social Science at the University of Plymouth. She also has a joint appointment in the Public Health Development Unit (Plymouth Teaching Primary Care Trust). Her current research interests include local public health issues, solo living, and individualisation.

David H. J. Morgan is Professor Emeritus in Sociology at the University of Manchester where he taught for approximately 35 years. He is currently Visiting Professor at Keele University and is working on the 'sociology of acquaintanceship'. One of his recent publications is *Transitions in Context* (with C. Holdsworth, Open University Press, 2005).

Chris Phillipson is Professor of Applied Social Studies and Social Gerontology at Keele University where he is also a Pro-Vice Chancellor. His most recent books are *The Futures of Old Age* (co-edited, Sage Books, 2006) and *Aging, Globalization and Inequality* (co-edited, Baywood Press, 2006). Present research includes work on an ESRC/AHRC-funded project examining the lives of the 'baby boom' generation.

Teresa Smith is University Lecturer in Social Policy and Social Work in the Department of Social Policy and Social Work, University of Oxford. Her research interests include community, family and childcare, parental involvement, and the evaluation of community-based programmes for young children and their families. She worked in the Educational Priority Areas projects in the late 1960s ('Whatever happened to EPAS?', 2007), studied parental participation in Oxfordshire preschools in the 1970s (*Parents and preschool*, 1980), published one of the earliest studies on family centres in the 1990s (*Family centres and bringing up young children*, 1996), and played a lead role in evaluation of the government's Neighbourhood Nurseries Initiative (*The Neighbourhood Nurseries Initiative National Evaluation: Final Integrated Report*, 2007). She is an advisor to the House of Commons Children, Schools and Families Select Committee.

Lawrence Ware is currently based in the Research and Innovation division of the University of Plymouth. Since gaining his PhD in 2002, he has been involved in several research projects that utilise large data sets. In addition to solo-living, these projects include studies of voting behaviour and non-response in local elections and issues surrounding migrant workers in South West England.

Jeffrey Weeks is University Director of Research and Director of SPUR (Social Policy and Urban Regeneration Research Institute) at London South Bank University. He has written widely on the history and social organisation of sexuality and intimate life, and is the author or editor of over twenty books and one hundred papers on related themes. Recent books include *Making Sexual History* (Polity Press, 2000), *Same Sex Intimacies* (with Brian Heaphy and Catherine Donovan, Routledge, 2001), *Sexualities and Society: A Reader* (co-edited with Janet Holland and Matthew Waites, Polity Press, 2003), and *The World We Have Won* (Routledge, 2007).

Malcolm Williams is Professor of Social Research Methodology at the University of Plymouth. His empirical research has been in the areas of migration, housing need, and households. Much of this work has used the ONS Longitudinal Study. His methodological publications are mainly in the area of scientific method in the social sciences.

Gail Wilson is Reader Emeritus in Social Policy and Ageing at the London School of Economics. Since 1987 she has researched and written about normal ageing in older men and women, especially those over the age of 75. Her main interest has been globalisation, with particular reference to gender, migration and identity in later life, access to health and social services, and qualitative research methods. She has published *Understanding Old Age: Critical and Global Perspectives* (Sage, 2000), *Community Care: Asking the Users* (edited collection, Chapman and Hall, 1995), and numerous academic- and practitioner-oriented articles.

Chapter 1

Introduction

Rosalind Edwards

Recent years have seen concerns expressed about the nature of transformations in family and community relationships, including how they are affected by and affect social and economic developments. But how can we think about and assess the nature of the present in relation to the past, and vice versa? What are the methodologies involved in enabling such assessments? This edited volume highlights an important area where knowledge can be contradictory and uncertain, in terms of the concepts employed to guide research and perspectives shaping understanding of family, community and generational change. Further, new methodologies are emerging alongside established ones in researching the topic.

This collection is organised around the two key themes of concepts and methodologies. Contributing authors look at these issues in relation to various aspects of family and community life over time, across generations. They are concerned, as Jeffrey Weeks neatly puts it in this volume, with 'the historic present and living past'. Contributions run from those addressing concepts and understanding trends, through those exploring concepts and the possibilities and practice of 'revisitation' study, to those looking at concepts and longitudinal large-scale data sets.

The time period covered is the latter half of the twentieth century and the beginning of the twenty-first century. This span encompasses a number of important social shifts. These shifts include the collectivisation of life risks through to the creation of the modern welfare state, followed more recently by the individualisation of life risks through their increasing privatisation and marketisation. Large-scale immigration has led to a plurality of cultures and affiliations. Sex and reproduction were further unhooked with the introduction of the pill as a reliable birth control method. There has been increasing diversity and fluidity in family forms, not least through rising rates of divorce, cohabitation and lone parenthood. Challenges to established gender relations have been bolstered by increasing numbers of women, especially mothers, entering the labour force. And the period of childhood has been extended as young people remain in education and are economically dependent (Brannen *et al.* 2004; Lewis 2007; Wadsworth *et al.* 2003). While the substance of the chapters is framed within the British context, the considerations of concepts and methodologies in exploring change have a wider relevance beyond the nationally specific.

This collection begins with reflective pieces by Graham Crow on discernment of levels of change and continuity in relation to communities over time; David H. J. Morgan on the contemporary potential of concepts developed in classic community studies of the late 1950s and 1960s, such as boundaries and identities; Jeffrey Weeks on shifts in the ways sexuality has been regulated and experienced since the mid-1940s; and Harry Goulbourne on recurring themes in how the integration of minority ethnic communities and families has been understood since the late 1960s.

Following on these conceptual and trend overviews and critiques, this volume continues by looking at revisitation research, either in terms of revisiting and re-analysing original data or revisiting and replicating previous studies. Quite often the studies revisited were themselves conducted in the context of a sense of being on the cusp of social change. In terms of revisitation through re-analysis, Val Gillies explores the knotty methodological issue of context in secondary analysis of available in-depth data from studies conducted in the 1960s in order to trace shifts in parenting resources over time. Joanna Bornat and Gail Wilson discuss the practice of, and findings concerning discourses about family from, a re-analysis of oral history interviews about the development of geriatric practice before and after the establishment of the National Health Service collected in the early 1990s. In terms of revisitation through replication, Chris Phillipson, and Nickie Charles and colleagues reflect on the methodological issues they faced in conducting contemporary versions of classic studies (which were conducted during the late 1940s and 1950s, and the early 1960s, respectively), involving both quantitative and qualitative analyses, and their findings on older people and on intergenerational family life from these endeavours.

The focus on various sorts of 'revisitation' methodology as part of attempts to research change over generations is followed by pieces on large-scale statistical data sets specifically concerned with tracking change in individual and family life over time. Denise Hawkes reviews long-standing and new cohort studies, with a particular focus on the potential of the recent UK Millennium Cohort Study illustrated by the example of early motherhood; and Malcolm Williams and colleagues assess the strengths and weaknesses of working with large-scale longitudinal data sets, specifically looking at solo living from the early 1970s. Finally, Teresa Smith turns to the concepts and investigations underpinning policies in reviewing interactions and shifts between ideas of community and notions of local area in identification of problems and interventions in the preschool field from the 1960s on.

Background to the collection

Before elaborating on the chapter contributions in conceptual and methodological context in this introduction, it is important to note that a volume such as this cannot cover all possible ways of exploring social change over generations. This is especially the case given the recent burgeoning of interest in charting changes and continuities in family and community life. Notably – although there is discussion of a recent large-scale survey data set that will be charting changes into the future (the Millennium Cohort Study) – as the collection was being put together a new initiative in the field of qualitative longitudinal research began: the 'Timescapes' study. This multi-project study will shed light on the dynamics of personal relationships over the life course into the future. Various small-scale qualitative projects following individuals over extended periods of time also exist (see review in Holland et al. 2006).

Further, this collection is missing one contribution in particular. The majority of the chapters have been developed from presentations as part of a series of seminars that was held in 2005–6. The seminar series was organised by the Families & Social Capital ESRC Research Group at London South Bank University in collaboration with the Academy of Learned Societies for the Social Sciences and funded by the Economic and Social Research Council. One important contribution to the series came from Professor Dennis Marsden, who unfortunately was not able to develop his paper into a chapter because of ill health. He is one of Britain's 'pioneers' of qualitative sociological research, conducting several classic studies in the 1960s and continuing to produce influential work into the new millennium (Thompson and Corti 2004).

Marsden's seminar paper reflected on whether or not two of his classic studies, *Education and the Working Class* (Jackson and Marsden 1962) and *Mothers Alone* (Marsden 1973), could either be repeated or the original data re-analysed. He pointed out that a variety of changes have made it increasingly difficult to replicate these studies of social class bias in education and the poverty of lone mothers in their original form. For example, there are now fewer grammar schools (albeit alongside new forms of educational selection), greater geographical mobility, fewer intact families, changed social security arrangements, tighter official control on granting access for research, and so on. Nevertheless, he felt that official statistics about the contemporary situation underline the continuing need for sensitive qualitative research into the issues identified in the original studies. For example, continued class gradients in education mandate further research focusing on selectivity. *Education and the Working Class* found a group differentiated along lines such as 'rough and respectable', but also a 'sunken middle class', and evidence that middle-class culture was not opened up to working-class grammar school boys. Marsden argued that research on education has continued to point to the need for awareness of the role that certain kinds of cultural and social capital play in gaining access to privilege and the reinforcement of social exclusion. Selectivity now operates in different, often hidden, ways including streaming in schools and the operation of parental choice and middle-class cultural capital.

Turning to archived data from his classic studies, Marsden argued that, rather than providing a raw resource for the research community, the material is inevitably personal and produced in context. He felt that such archived data would perhaps be better understood with the help of a detailed commentary by the researchers involved, giving their account of the conception, context, processing, and production of the data for the final report. Interviews were not audio-recorded in the classic studies, so the archived material constitutes a three-level filter between the original individual accounts given during interviews, the data 'recovered' from the interviews, and the final publication. Finally, Marsden called for the reappearance of social class in policy as well as academic discussion, alongside greater government appreciation of small-scale qualitative studies.

Marsden's discussion thus touched on recurring and common themes in the contributions to this edited collection. Such themes include issues of changing social and political context, as well as some crucial continuities, and the importance of acknowledging the perspectives that shape researching family, community, and generational change.

Family and community across generations

The definitions and meanings of 'family' and 'community' are contested, as is the relationship between them. The terms conceptually shift over time and in their understanding of the constitution of everyday life.

A functional concept of family puts an emphasis on the structure of families and the structure of the roles undertaken by its members, creating an adaptive fit between families and the societies in which they are located. Thus 'family' is about the production of new members of society, their socialisation into society's culture, and their everyday maintenance – with some family forms, notably the nuclear family, seen as most fit for these responsibilities (see discussion in Charles and colleagues' chapter). In contrast, alternative conceptions of family have recently been concerned not with a static category or structure, but with a more dynamic understanding of family as diverse in a complex and fluid society. Family is said to have become disassociated from prescribed kin relations and roles, and more associated with individualised and contingent personal, intimate relationships. People, it is argued, create their own sorts of relationships and commitments in the endlessly fluid form of what some have called 'families of choice', rather than following handed-down, unquestioned and permanent roles and obligations (e.g. Giddens 1992; Weeks *et al.* 2001).

A similar trajectory, from stasis to fluidity, is evident for the concept of 'community'. Community as a body of people who are conscious of having something in common, leading to a sense of shared interests, identity, and solidarity, has traditionally been thought of as integrally situated in local geographical context. While this understanding of where community is located continues, there are also arguments that these local supports and homogeneous groups are eroding, marked by disruption and contingency. Community is said to have become 'disembedded' and lifted out of social relations in a particular location (e.g. Giddens 1990). Rather, the form of those social relations is now envisaged as fragmenting and proliferating into a variety of 'symbolic' or 'imagined' communities, personal communities of interest and attachment, and virtual communities (e.g. Anderson 1993; Bauman 1998; Cohen 1985).

Traditionally, there has been a close conceptual relationship between family-as-kinship and community-as-locality; families are part of the constitution of communities, and communities form a context for living family life. These interpenetrations provided a link between the individual and the larger social structures (see Driver and Martell 2002 on policy linkage). Classic community studies, such as those discussed by Crow and Morgan, and those revisited by Phillipson, are often interwoven with accounts of family life, and vice versa, as in the revisitation by Charles and colleagues. The recent unhooking of family from blood and law, and of community from locality, however, has problematised the relationship between the two – family may be tangential to what is considered 'community' in contemporary individualised and globalised society.

The concept of generation is also bound up in this, as change is often understood as the dynamics of the sequence of generations. As individual members of families move through the life course, are born, grow older and die, new families are formed and the communities of which they are part are socially reproduced. On the one hand, these generational dynamics are understood as a source of stability over time, in providing links between the past and present and the 'handing down' of social mores. On the other hand, they are viewed as a major engine of change over time as established and 'handed down' practices and values are revised and reshaped or overturned and ousted by new ones.

Perspectives on change and continuity

The idea of change over generations – rather than attention to continuity – has become a preoccupation of the contemporary focus on family and community life. Debates about families and communities are largely structured around the premise that social and economic changes have influenced and/or been driven by changes in the way people relate to each other, and that the state of families and communities are connected (Gillies 2003).

There are two dominant perspectives on such changes, both often citing the same data about families and communities, but with quite different implications. One perspective sees a breakdown of established social ties and cohesion (e.g. Coleman 1990; Davies 1993; Dennis and Erdos 1992; Etzioni 1993; Fevre 2000; Murray 1994; Putnam 1993, 2000). The other perspective suggests that greater diversity and plurality of populations and lifestyles generates new opportunities for democratic and reciprocal relations (e.g. Beck and Beck-Gernsheim 1995, 2002; Giddens 1991, 1992; Stacey 1996; Weeks 1995; Weeks *et al.* 2001). The 1960s are often identified in both these perspectives as the historical point at which either decline or renewal began to take hold. Thus the field has become positioned around a somewhat polarised framework for understanding family, community, and generational change.

A third perspective, however, questions the extent of demise or regeneration in family and community life (e.g. Crow 2000; Jamieson 1998). There are arguments that a preoccupation with documenting change means that cyclical patterns are mistaken for linear transformations (Stanley 1992), and that social divisions cutting across families and communities may have been 'disembedded' but there is a form of continuity in that they then become 're-embedded' in revised ways (Adkins 2002). Moreover, as indicated earlier, as concepts, both family and community may have quite different, or even contradictory, meanings within a given time period as well as across time (e.g. Anderson 1993). And notions of change usually speak to contemporary concerns, retelling the past in relation to the present, and constituting the present through differences between a remembered past and images of the future (Adam 2004; Zerubavel 2003).

Debates about linear progression, functionalist adaptation, turning points, or cycles of growth and decay have long characterised discussions of social change generally, and it is evident that whether or not change is identified is dependent on the standpoint of observation. The approaches taken in this volume, mainly focusing on looking back in order to understand the present, vividly illustrate the importance of aspect and context in making substantive judgements about the trajectory of family and community life across generations, integrally allied to the perspectives provided by the concepts and methodologies that researchers utilise.

Continuity alongside change is evident across and within the range of chapter contributions, and in turn this highlights the importance of the aspect of families and communities under consideration. For example, in looking at sexuality then it may be possible, as Weeks argues, to discern a world of new possibilities since the mid-1940s, albeit with some enduring 'downsides'. When it comes to minority ethnic families in Britain, however, while there has been change in relation to increasing diversity, Goulbourne's analysis is that there appears to be old wine from the 1970s in the contemporary bottles of concern about possibilities for integration – an analysis which is echoed more generally in Smith's discussion of linguistic shifts from 'community' as the lever for intervention to that of 'area'. More generally, Morgan points out that past community studies show that boundaries and identities are fundamental and recurrent negotiated motifs in how people understand their communities and reveal that diversity and division has long been associated with community – whether localised, personal or virtual. For him, this highlights the contribution that the particular can make to understanding the general, where specific place-based community studies can illuminate wider issues concerning stability and change. Continuity alongside change is also evident in post-war family and community ties. Charles and colleagues demonstrate the way that kinship ties for family members show both increased social and cultural differentiation related to economic differentiation as well as continued characterisation by locality and gender, while Phillipson discusses the way kinship ties for older people remain evident but personal social ties have become more significant. Smith also points to variability in continuity or decline when it comes to studies looking at community cohesion and social capital across time.

Policies are introduced by governments with the intention of bringing about change and, indeed, legal contexts can shift, as Weeks discusses in relation to sexuality. Nonetheless, policies are also built on previous developments, initiatives, and modifications. This co-existence of continuity alongside change draws attention to methods of investigation.

Taken on a purely practical level, changed data collection contexts on the structural level can pose problems in making direct comparison between past and present. For example, Charles and colleagues draw attention to difficulties posed by administrative boundary and population changes in their Swansea-based re-study, as well as the way that replication of the original questionnaire had to be modified because of the changed empirical and theoretical context. While Charles and colleagues thus worked with and made this aspect of replication explicit, Phillipson's way of handling these difficulties was to work with broad findings from the original studies and adopt different methods to illuminate them in the contemporary context. With respect to large-scale data sets, Williams and colleagues refer to changes in the construction of questions, and thus variables, between data collection points in longitudinal statistical research, while Hawkes demonstrates the significance of different levels of geographical analysis within a longitudinal data set. Related to this point about levels, Crow points out that a focus on individuals highlights change, while a focus on structures and resources often illuminates continuities.

Whatever the difficulties though – as many of the contributors to this volume stress – working with situated empirical data cannot be jettisoned in favour of making 'grand narrative' judgements about family, community, and generational change. They also note how mixed methods can bring strength to this endeavour. Quantitative data that regularly charts what is changing over time overcomes the issue of discrete snapshots and is complemented by the insights into how practices are changing or enduring provided by qualitative data (Holland *et al.* 2006).

As well as the methods of comparison, the perspectives which are adopted can lead to the privileging of some evidence and the downplaying of other evidence. Charles and colleagues warn that adopting past conceptual frameworks and definitions can privilege continuity at the expense of change – and the point can also be made vice versa. As both Crow and Gillies point out, as well as the substantive object of scrutiny, research frameworks and agendas can change over time in terms of what is seen as significant. Indeed, as Gillies also argues, no data is neutral and re-analysing or replicating researchers need to be aware of both the historic and contemporary social contexts of their production. Gillies and Bornat and Wilson regard secondary analysis in particular as a 're-making' of new data rather than a straightforward accessing of original material. All of these points about what is being seen through what lens are clearly demonstrated in Bornat and Wilson's discussion of pursuing issues concerning community, family, and ethnicity that were 'silent' in the original research focus. These points are also demonstrated in Phillipson's remarks on how older people's personal communities may not have been less significant in the past but merely not a focus of past studies, while more current theoretical lenses highlight them. Further, how research agendas might intersect with political agendas is raised by both Hawkes' description of the foci of previous and new cohort studies, and Smith's discussion of the transformation of community into area-based intervention policy initiatives.

Overall, then, this collection demonstrates the conceptual and methodological range and complexity involved in the endeavour of looking back – and therefore also of tracking forward – in order to understand transformations and continuities in family and community lives over generations.

References

Adam, B. (2004) *Time*, Oxford: Blackwell.
Adkins, L. (2002) *Revisions: Gender and Sexuality in Late Modernity*, Milton Keynes: Open University Press.
Anderson B (1993) *Imagined Communities*, London: Verso.
Bauman, Z. (1998) *Globalization*, Cambridge: Polity Press.
Beck, U. and Beck-Gernsheim, E. (1995) *The Normal Chaos of Love*, Cambridge: Polity Press.
Beck, U. and Beck-Gernsheim, E. (2002) *Individualisation*, London: Sage.
Brannen, J., Moss, P. and Mooney, A. (2004) *Working and Caring over the Twentieth Century: Change and Continuity in Four-Generation Families*, Basingstoke: Palgrave.
Cohen, A. (1985) *The Symbolic Construction of Community*, London: Routledge.
Coleman, J.S. (1990) *Foundations of Social Theory*, London: Harvard University Press.

Crow, G. (2000) *Social Solidarities: Theories, Identities and Social Change*, Buckingham: Open University Press.

Davies, J. (1993) *The Family: Is It Just Another Lifestyle Choice?*, London: Institute for Economic Affairs.

Dennis, N. and Erdos, G. (1992) *Families Without Fatherhood*, London: Institute for Economic Affairs.

Driver, S. and Martell, L. (2002) 'New Labour, work and the family', *Social Policy and Administration*, 36(1): 46–61.

Etzioni, A. (1993) *The Parenting Deficit*, London: Demos.

Fevre, R. (2000) *The Demoralisation of Western Culture*, London: Continuum.

Giddens, A. (1990) *The Consequences of Modernity*, Cambridge: Polity Press.

Giddens, A. (1991) *Modernity and Self-Identity: Self and Society in the Late Modern Age*, Cambridge: Polity Press.

Giddens, A. (1992) *The Transformation of Intimacy: Sexuality, Love and Eroticism in Modern Societies*, Cambridge: Polity Press.

Gillies, V. (2003) *Family and Intimate Relationships: A Review of the Sociological Literature*, Families & Social Capital ESRC Research Group Working Paper No. 2, London: London South Bank University.

Holland, J., Thomson, R. and Henderson, S. (2006) *Qualitative Longitudinal Research: A Discussion Paper*, Families & Social Capital ESRC Research Group Working Paper No. 21, London: London South Bank University.

Jackson, B. and Marsden, D. (1962) *Education and the Working Class: Some General Themes Raised by a Study of 88 Working Class Children*, London: Routledge and Kegan Paul.

Jamieson, L. (1998) *Intimacy: Personal Relationships in Modern Societies*, Cambridge: Polity Press.

Lewis, J. (ed.) (2007) *Children, Changing Families and Welfare States*, Cheltenham: Edward Elgar.

Marsden, D. (1973) *Mothers Alone: Poverty and the Fatherless Family*, London: Penguin.

Murray, C. (1994) *Underclass: The Crisis Deepens*, London: IEA Health and Welfare Unit.

Putnam, R.D. (1993) *Making Democracy Work: Civic Traditions in Modern Italy*, Princeton: Princeton University Press.

Putnam, R.D. (2000) *Bowling Alone: The Collapse and Revival of American Community*, New York: Simon and Schuster.

Stacey, J. (1996) *In the Name of the Family: Rethinking Family Values in the Postmodern Age*, Boston: Beacon Press.

Stanley, L. (1992) 'Changing households, changing work', in N. Abercrombie and A. Ward (eds) *Social Change in Contemporary Britain*, Cambridge: Polity Press.

Thompson, P. and Corti, L. (eds) (2004) 'Celebrating Classic Sociology: Pioneers of Contemporary British Qualitative Research', Special Issue, *International Journal of Social Research Methodology: Theory and Practice*, 7(1).

Wadsworth, M., Ferri, E. and Bynner, J. (2003) 'Changing Britain', in E. Ferri, J. Bynner and M. Wadsworth (eds) *Changing Britain, Changing Lives: Three Generations at the Turn of the Century*, Bedford Way Papers, London: Institute of Education, University of London.

Weeks, J. (1995) *Invented Moralities: Sexual Values in an Age of Uncertainty*, New York: Columbia University Press.

Weeks, J., Donovan, C. and Heaphy, B. (2001) *Same Sex Intimacies: Families of Choice and Other Life Experiments*, London: Routledge.

Zerubavel, E. (2003) *Time Maps: Collective Memory and the Social Space of the Past*, Chicago: Chicago University Press.

Chapter 2

Thinking about families and communities over time

Graham Crow

Introduction

Towards the end of his life Karl Marx remarked that 'To save the Russian commune a Russian revolution will be necessary' (in Nicolaievsky and Maenchen-Helfen 1976: 422). This is one of several social scientific paradoxes that take the form of identifying that things need to change if things are to stay the same (Crow 2005). Community and family relationships are prominent among these demonstrations of how analysis in terms of a simple opposition between *either* continuity *or* change has serious limitations, because continuity and change are often to be found together. It has long been recognised that the reproduction of patterns of family relationships involves frequent adjustment to change by the individuals who participate in them, for example the reworking of the ties between family members of different generations as they age. Families work towards children becoming more independent and setting up their own households in order that they can continue to function as supportive family or kin networks. Leaving home is thus a time of change and continuity: 'material and emotional support for children at this time of *household* disruption is a means by which *family* solidarities can be sustained despite the changes occurring' (Allan and Crow 2001: 44, emphases in original). Another illustration of this point about things changing in order for things to stay the same is Bill Williams' notion of 'dynamic equilibrium' in his study of the adjustment of farming families to the variations in their needs and capabilities over the course of what used to be called the life cycle. These farming families expanded or contracted their land holdings according to the availability of family labour on which they could draw, with the result that 'the social structure *as a whole* appears relatively unchanged and unchanging' (Williams 1963: xviii, emphasis in original). At the same time, individual families and their members could undergo dramatic changes of fortune involving upward or downward social mobility.

Williams was prompted to undertake his research by other people's attachment to what he regarded as a conception of community which was too 'neat and tidy'. He was puzzled by what he described as 'a strange reluctance to abandon the notion of the unchanging, traditional countryside' (Williams 1963: xvii–xviii) that was rooted in Ferdinand Tönnies's nineteenth-century account of *gemeinschaft*. Many other writers have made similar points about this and related conceptual frameworks surviving well beyond the point when they cease to be analytically useful. In the study of family relationships, for example, Judith Stacey's critique of conventional accounts argues that real families are 'much more complex and contradictory' (Stacey 1998: xiii) than the nuclear family norm which they promote. This is an important element in her argument that it is appropriate to regard domestic arrangements that deviate from this norm as different types of families – in her terms as *Brave New Families*. Another way of expressing this idea is Elisabeth Beck-Gernsheim's comment that 'The answer to the question "What next after the family?" is ... quite simple: the family'; more precisely it is the 'post-familial family' (Beck-Gernsheim 2002: ix). For the same reasons, new forms of community are still usefully thought of as communities, rather than accepting the view that the passing of traditional communities marks the death of community as such. The two crucial general points to emphasise are that communities and families are much better understood as dynamic rather than static entities, and that change over time is producing further diversity rather than moving things towards any one type of arrangement. There are, in other words, good reasons why we now tend to refer to 'families' rather than 'the family' and 'communities' rather than 'the community'. This allows for the range of family and community forms and practices to be acknowledged, and for universal claims about any one family or community form to be challenged. It also allows the temporal dimension of family and community relationships to be opened up so that these relationships are understood less as static and fixed arrangements and more as dynamic and fluid. Within this developing conceptual framework, it is possible to account for the paradoxical co-existence of continuity and change.

The co-existence of continuity and change

The co-existence of continuity and change is a well-established theme in the literature on communities. Margaret Stacey's two studies of Banbury highlight this theme in their titles: *Tradition and Change* (Stacey 1960) and *Power, Persistence and Change* (Stacey et al. 1975). Stacey concluded the first of these studies with the observation that 'the traditional and the non-traditional constantly interact' (Stacey 1960: 182), and argued that this was particularly noticeable in the realm of values in which new forms of traditionalism could be seen to be evolving. The second study confirmed the expectation that in terms of social norms and values, further significant change had occurred in the interim, but it also threw up the finding that in the distribution of power and resources 'marked inequalities ... appear remarkably persistent' (Stacey et al. 1975: 132–3). At the individual level it could seem to Banburians that change was endemic, as the arrival of large numbers of migrants to the town and other external influences made the old order impossible to sustain, but at a more structural level the town continued to be 'an ordered society' (Stacey *et al.* 1975: 135). The discovery of more continuity than researchers at the outset expected to find is a feature of many other studies – from Michael Young and Peter Willmott's (1957) classic *Family and Kinship in East London* (in which working-class kinship networks were treated as unexpectedly resilient in the context of the development of the welfare state) to Tim Butler and Garry Robson's (2003) discovery of the remarkable persistence and pervasiveness among middle-class gentrifiers of commitment to living among others like themselves, captured in their frequently-expressed endorsement of 'people like us' (Crow 2004). A parallel to this latter case is provided by Mike Savage and his colleagues' (2005) discovery of a strong commitment to 'ordinariness' among the middle-class residents of greater Manchester whom they interviewed, which stands in contrast to the common-sense expectation that upward mobility prompts the development of a more individualised outlook in which local community-mindedness necessarily plays only a limited role.

The solution to the paradox of continuity and change co-existing may thus be no more complicated than the observation that one element of community life may stay the same despite another element changing. Community relationships do not constitute a single, integrated and indivisible whole in which one part changing means that everything else must change as well. Changes in the values held by residents of Banbury were quite consistent with the reproduction of inequalities in power and life chances among those same residents; indeed, the 'modernisation' of 'traditional' legitimisations of inequality in all probability contributed to the prospects of these inequalities being sustainable. Conversely, changes in people's material circumstances and life chances, such as those accompanying the development of the welfare state or those associated with geographical and social mobility, do not necessarily involve abandonment of previously held values and identities. Precisely the same points can be made about family relationships witnessing 'the intertwining of change and continuity' (McRae 1999: 19). Contemporary ideals of the relationship between partners and also between parents and children emphasise the shift from obligation to choice and from hierarchy to equality, but Lynn Jamieson has noted that elements of continuity make it doubtful 'that this picture of change sums up how people are behaving towards each other in practice' (Jamieson 1998: 161). Carol Smart and Bren Neale (1999) have argued along similar lines that gender inequalities in childcare responsibilities and access to resources have the potential to survive changes in family ideals and their embodiment in new legal codes. On the other hand, significant change in patterns of household composition does not necessarily mean that established conceptions of family life are jettisoned. Among the step-families interviewed by Jacqueline Burgoyne and David Clark (1984), the majority sought to achieve 'ordinary' family life, and only a minority saw themselves as pioneers of a new family form. Jane Ribbens McCarthy and her co-authors report a similar finding from their research among step-families, whose members typically rejected '"step-family" as a term that applied to their own ... situation' (Ribbens McCarthy et al. 2003: 23). In their view the term wrongly emphasised their distinctiveness rather than their normality as families.

If change in the realm of values relating to families and communities is compatible with continuities in important aspects of how families and communities operate in practice, and if the converse situation also applies to change in family and community practices being consistent with continuities in the realm of values and ideals, then a challenge exists regarding how we think about what constitutes continuity and what counts as change. Simple models that represent past arrangements as traditional and contrast this with an image of wholesale change in which these arrangements have been swept away are inadequate, for all their superficial persuasiveness. Zygmunt Bauman, for example, claims that

'community' stands for the kind of world which is not, regrettably, available to us' because we now 'live in ruthless times ... when people around seem to keep their cards close to their chests and few people seem in any hurry to help us

(Bauman 2001: 3)

In the same vein, Ulrich Beck has asserted that 'community is dissolved in the acid bath of competition' (Beck 1992: 94). Accounts of contemporary arrangements that are empirically grounded present a picture that is much more nuanced than such sweeping speculative assessments are able to achieve. Studies of virtual communities, for example, consistently reveal that although they are the antithesis of 'traditional' place-based communities in terms of their ability to escape the constraints of face-to-face interaction, they remain reliant for their functioning on adherence to norms of group behaviour and a sense of collective identity (Hornsby 1998). Technology on its own does not change communities any more than it does families, as research into the impact of technological change on the domestic division of labour has shown (Gershuny 2000). Understanding the interconnections of continuity and change requires something more than an emphasis on an overarching theme, whether that chosen theme is individualisation, democratisation or one of a number of other possibilities.

Reframing continuity and change

Gershuny's research into changing patterns of people's time use reminds us that the purpose of investigations into this issue is not only to produce an account of the greater or lesser extent of change but also to furnish an explanation that will stand up to scrutiny. In Gershuny's case, what he is seeking to explain (changing time use in economic and social life) is clear and the longitudinal data on which he draws provide a basis for confidence that what is being compared over time is more or less the same entity. This is not an assumption that holds good for all research methods. In community re-studies, for example, the purpose of researchers going back to a place that has been investigated previously is to capture continuity and change over the intervening period, but the research agenda as well as the object of the research require scrutiny in this respect. Commenting on the comparison of the findings of the second Banbury study with those of the first, Colin Bell identified this as the problem of separating out 'social change' from 'socio-logical change' (Bell 1977: 60). The second study differed from the first not only because the town and its people had changed but also because the ideas informing the research team had evolved – particularly because of Stacey's move away from the search for 'community' and its associated mythology. Bell was, of course, mindful of how this issue had been raised by the classic 1930s re-study of 'Middletown' by Robert and Helen Lynd which was 'markedly different in tone' (Bell and Newby 1971: 84) from the original study conducted by the Lynds in the previous decade, and which could be considered to have resulted (in part at least) from their reading of Marx in the interim. There is unmistakably far more emphasis on the power that accrues to wealth holders in the second volume than there was in the first.

The town of Muncie, Indiana (where the 'Middletown' studies were conducted) has been the subject of extensive research ever since, and the recent investigation by Luke Lassiter and his associates provides a further illustration of how more recent publications can reflect not only social change but also change in the way in which research problems are framed. The Lynds deliberately bracketed out 'racial change' from their agenda in order to concentrate more effectively on 'cultural change' (Lynd and Lynd 1929: 8), and their exclusion of the town's small but nevertheless signifi-cant African-American population was continued until the work undertaken by Lassiter and his team righted that omission (Lassiter *et al.* 2004). Another re-study in which the account of social change and the impact of sociological change are hard to disentangle is Lois Bryson's return to 'Newtown' in suburban Australia in the 1990s, two decades on from her original study. In the original study (Bryson and Thompson 1972) 'gender was not explicitly discussed as a fundamental cleavage of social relations'. The re-study, conducted in the light of the development of feminist analyses, provided 'an opportunity to reconsider women's posi-tion' from a new vantage point (Bryson and Winter 1999: 15). This evolution of perspective did not prevent the re-study setting out 'to explore change and continuity in the decades leading up to the end of the twentieth century' (Bryson and Winter 1999: 207). The finding that economic inequalities had become more marked was a major element of change, yet this was compatible with the observation that 'In terms of social interaction with family, friends and neighbours, the patterns in the 1990s had much in common with those in the 1960s' (Bryson and Winter 1999: 213). In very broad terms, this report is the opposite of the patterns of change and continuity discerned by Stacey and her colleagues between the two Banbury studies.

In some cases the provision by an original study of a benchmark against which subsequent change can be gauged is complicated by an emphasis on change already underway. The original research on Swansea published as *The Family and Social Change* described a situation of emergent patterns of social and geographical mobility as things moved from 'the cohesive society' (or, less flatteringly, 'the stagnant society') to 'the mobile society' (Rosser and Harris 1965: 299). The re-study by Charlotte Aull Davies and Nickie Charles forty years on is in some ways engaged in reporting on continuing change along these lines and the complication of this pattern by other trends such as the growing ethnic diversity of the town's population and 'the proliferation of family and household types' (Davies and Charles 2002: 2.1). The inclusion in the original study of quantitative as well as qualitative data allows comparison with the situation in the half-century up to 1960 whereby only 42 per cent of couples started out married life in a home on their own, while 50 per cent lived initially with either the wife's or the husband's parents, and the remaining 8 per cent lived with other relatives (Rosser and Harris 1965: 250). This situation is surprising enough in itself, given twenty-first century understandings of the normality of 'a home of one's own', but the detailed figures reveal a further surprise in that the percentage of couples starting out married life in a home on their own actually *decreased* from 52 per cent in the first part of this period to 31 per cent in the latter decades of 1940–60. Likewise, the continued existence of enforced residence with parents should not be thought to have disappeared with the passage of time, at least not in all areas. (See Chapter 8 for further discussion of the *Families and Social Change* re-study.) Anthea Holme's study of young families in East London following the birth of a first child found 17 per cent of them living as part of another household, and they were disproportionately located in the poorer of the two areas studied where a higher proportion of the mothers were single parents (Holme 1985: 180). There is, in other words, a much more complicated story to tell than a simple linear process of growth in nuclear families occupying a home of their own.

Theorising continuity and change

Holme's explanation of the patterns that she found highlights the contrasts that accompany processes of social polarisation, and in doing so she draws on an established mode of thinking in terms of centrifugal and centripetal forces which propel some people to the periphery while others are bound close to the centre. In geographical terms, 'centrifugal population movement' takes families to suburban accommodation that is more spacious, attractive and owner-occupied while inner-city life is exemplified by the young single mother who 'lives with her parents in a grim block of council flats' (Holme 1985: 159–60). In this geographical understanding of centrifugal forces, Holme follows Young and Willmott's (1975: 38) lead, but other analyses use the idea of centrifugal and centripetal forces to convey the notion of people being propelled to the social margins or pulled towards the centre of social relationships. Dennis Warwick and Gary Littlejohn, for example, argue that such an analysis helps to explain change and continuity in communities being brought about by 'forces beyond the control of individual members and households' and illuminates how these processes may 'be marked with contradictions and tensions' (Warwick and Littlejohn 1992: 20). It is certainly possible to see the various macro-level forces that have been identified in the literature as driving change in family and community life as ones that are in tension with each other. This is particularly so if the shifts of themes in this literature are acknowledged, from Maurice Stein's (1964) emphasis on the three key movements of urbanisation, industrialisation and bureaucratisation to the proliferation of forces identified subsequently, including those that run counter to Stein's, such as counter-urbanisation and de-industrialisation (Crow 2002a).

A good example of bold theorising about family and community dynamics which subsequent developments and critiques have revealed to be unsustainable is Young and Willmott's notion of 'the slow march' whereby innovations are developed by one social group and spread over time as other social groups adopt them. Their argument is that 'many social changes start at the top and work downwards', and although they acknowledge that change 'downwards from the top to the bottom of the class structure' is not the only pattern, 'trickle down' (Young and Willmott 1975: 33, 27) is the predominant image on which they draw. Three main objections can be raised against the thesis that family and community change occurs in this way. The first objection is that change that starts at the bottom deserves more credit than it is given in such accounts. Judith Stacey's argument is that economic necessity rather than the existence of opportunity to innovate is what lies behind family change. In her view, 'African-American women and white, working-class women have been the genuine postmodern family pioneers' and she attaches particular importance to 'economic pressures' in her account of 'these departures from domesticity' (Stacey 1998: 252). Several other studies have suggested similar conclusions about innovations in household strategies emerging out of the need to respond to economic constraints among low-income groups – for example, what Ray Pahl calls 'survival strategies of the poor' (Pahl 1984: 317). The emergence of new community practices of mutual aid out of the difficult circumstances of a strike by members of an occupational community offers another illustration of this point (Crow 2002b: Chapter 4).

The second objection to the idea of a 'slow march' is that not everyone is necessarily marching in the same direction in search of the same objectives. In the context of social polarisation, a more plausible perspective is one in which groups move in different directions in terms of their social situations. Social polarisation may have a geographical expression – as in Holme's contrast between London's affluent suburbs and its impoverished inner-city areas – but Pahl's research on the Isle of Sheppey noted that it is quite possible for polarisation to 'affect next-door neighbours' (Pahl 1984: 309). The result is that a work-rich household and a work-poor household spatially exist side by side but in social terms they live in different worlds and move further apart. In Pahl's case this outcome arose from the uneven impact of de-industrialisation, but in the case of the impact of gentrification on inner-city communities, other driving forces are involved. Butler and Robson's argument is that the middle-class gentrifiers of various parts of inner-London have moved there to escape from the suburban locations where they were brought up, because 'the inner city provided the excitement and cultural buzz that had been so lacking in many of their childhoods' (Butler and Robson 2003: 163). In seeking proximity to heterogeneous inner-city urban villages they are reversing the pattern of their parents whose move to the suburbs Young and Willmott had charted. The same conclusion about diverse directions of travel can be drawn from Savage and his colleagues' (2005) research in the Manchester area, where the four localities in which interviews were conducted represent four very different lifestyles among which middle-class people can exercise a degree of choice. Stacey makes the more general point in relation to families that contemporary developments are towards 'a multiplicity of family and household arrangements'. As a result what is emerging is 'not a new model of family life, not the next stage in an orderly progression of family history, but the stage when the belief in a logical progression of stages breaks down' (Stacey 1998: 17, 18) because these developments are at odds with the progressive model's notion of movement in one direction.

Stacey's further comment that what is being witnessed is a movement 'backward to the postmodern family' (Stacey 1998: 251) directs attention to the third objection to the idea of a slow march, namely its association with linear conceptions of time. Michael Young (1988) himself came to question the value of concentrating attention on linear conceptions of time, arguing that there is a rhythmic and cyclical quality to many aspects of society and that the role of cyclical movements in the maintenance of continuity deserves to be accorded as much weight as the role of linear movements in effecting change. The logic of this argument leads, as Young acknowledged, to the need to re-evaluate how historical knowledge is treated in sociological analyses of the present, because once the assumption of time being linear is questioned it follows that historical materials that appear to reveal changes may also reveal continuities over the full course of a cycle. Tamara

Hareven's work on the history of the family raises the ensuing question of whether family structures that vary over the lifetime of their members while exhibiting important intergenerational continuities are better captured by the language of continuity or change – to which her answer is 'continuity and change'. Thus 'Individuals living in nuclear households at one time in their lives were likely to live in households containing extended kin or non-relatives at other times', but what at the individual level is experienced as change may be understood at the level of the household as the cyclical reproduction of a pattern. The conclusions about the balance of continuity and change thus depends on whether the perspective of 'individual time' or 'family time' (Hareven 2000: Pt 1, 13, 4) is adopted, or whether an analytical frame is adopted that has the capacity to integrate the two.

Conclusion

Three implications of these discussions about continuity and change are worth highlighting. The first implication is that researchers' decisions about the level at which their analysis is pitched will have important implications for their conclusions about whether continuity or change has greater prominence. There is not necessarily a contradiction between Geoff Dench and his colleagues in their re-study of *Family and Kinship in East London*, which says that 'ethnic division and competition is ... a recurring feature of East End life' and which notes a few sentences later that, in contrast with the 1950s when the original study had been undertaken, 'the situation had changed entirely by the 1990s', before going on to remark that 'Bangladeshi families today have lives that evoke, in some ways, those of the post-war Bethnal Greeners described by Young and Willmott' (Dench *et al.* 2006: 2–3). The people living in a community may be succeeded by others who nevertheless reproduce familiar patterns of relationships. Katherine Mumford and Anne Power's research in the same area concludes that rapid shifts in population composition are quite consistent with sustained 'attachment to community' (Mumford and Power 2003: 265), while Janet Foster's (1999) study of London's Docklands strikes a similar balance between the account of economic and demographic transformation of the area as expressions of globalisation and the acknowledgement of continuities expressed in the reproduction of strong notions of belonging and of community insiders and outsiders. This pattern of change experienced at the individual level and more macro-level continuities is reversed in Elizabeth Roberts' account of early twentieth-century women's lives in which she notes that 'In the period before 1940, despite the changes in family size and standards of living ... one is left with a sense of continuity in the lives of working-class women, centred on their homes, families and neighbourhoods' (Roberts 1984: 202–3). Suzanne Keller's remark that the study of community 'requires time and deep acquaintance to distill wheat from chaff, the enduring from the ephemeral' (Keller 2003: xiii) is apposite here, because the overall emphasis in any account will depend on the extent to which particular expressions of continuity and change are classified as fundamental or superficial, and acquiring the ability to gauge this is necessarily a lengthy process.

This leads on to the second, methodological implication of attempting to capture continuity and change. The three decades and more spent by Keller on researching the new community of Twin Rivers is a long time even by the standards of community studies, among which there are many examples of projects taking a decade or more to complete (Crow 2000: 181), but the underlying rationale is that only through data collection over time can the shortcomings of 'one-shot reconstructions of community' that miss 'the long-range view' (Keller 2003: 74, 8) be avoided. Longitudinal research undertaken from the outset specifically for the purpose of collecting data that are comparable over time produces the most reliable results but it is inevitably slow at producing results. Re-studies of original investigations offer a potential route to quicker results, but if they are undertaken as two snapshots with no easy access to the social processes at work in the intervening period then their findings need to be treated with appropriate caution, given that these processes may be more cyclical than linear in character. In addition, re-studies do not always operate with precisely the same agenda as that which informed the original, particularly if they are undertaken by different researchers. Other challenges arise when comparisons are made between the present and the past in areas where only generalised impressions about 'traditional' family and community arrangements are available. That such impressions can be unreliable has been amply demonstrated by studies using oral history techniques that have revealed great variations in family and community life in earlier generations, even between neighbouring populations such as the textile workers and women in more casual employment studied by Miriam Glucksmann. Her work reveals that patterns of social and economic life in Lancashire between the 1930s and 1970s by no means conformed to a single standard, and that what was traditional in one area could be quite different from the next. There was a distinct localism to these cultures, with contrasting understandings of life framed by notions of 'What it's like round here' (Glucksmann 2000: 146). Such findings cast serious doubt on arguments about continuity and change that are based on broad generalisations about traditional working-class family and community life in this and previous periods.

The third implication is that analyses of continuity and change can be framed in ways that are more or less positive or negative about these processes. In the discussion of change, reference to 'the slow march' of developments in family and community relationships conveys an imagery of progress that is absent from accounts which highlight loss and invoke nostalgia. And in the discussion of continuity, Nancy Scheper-Hughes has noted how the maintenance of tradition has tended to be negatively cast as 'stubborn conservatism, resistance to new ideas and techniques, and suspiciousness of outsiders' (Scheper-Hughes 2001: 301), but she goes on to argue that its psychological advantages for those under pressure to change should not be discounted. There are also connotations of the language used to describe the processes by which continuity and change come about. References to overarching trends such as de-industrialisation can have far-reaching consequences for the understanding of how change is brought about and how this understanding is acted upon. Peter Marris has argued that structural explanations of community change have a tendency to make people feel 'at a loss what to do' (Marris 1987: 2), because the forces described appear beyond control. Conversely, other concepts convey a sense of individuals having opportunities to exercise a degree of control in their lives. Janet Finch and Jennifer Mason's adoption of the concept of negotiation was made mindful of the fact that it 'emphasises that individuals do have some room for manoeuvre' (Finch and Mason 1993: 60). The same point can be made about individuals and households and the concept of strategy (Allan and Crow 2001: 203).

In other words, the analysis of continuity and change necessarily involves discussion of the central sociological issue of structure and agency. This point is captured nicely in David Cheal's account of what he calls 'situational diversity', in which he takes the examples of migrants living alone and apart from their families to illustrate that 'people with the same cultural ideals of family life may live in different ways because practical circumstances affect the choices they make' (Cheal 2002: 27). In his earlier work (and acknowledging the influence of Katja Boh), Cheal had already flagged up the paradoxical character of growing diversity in family forms, noting that as movement towards '*destandardisation* of the family' spreads and is recognised, so we can identify a process of '*convergence to diversity*' (Cheal 1991: 133, 125, emphases in original) in the patterns of family life that are nevertheless still recognisable as 'family practices' (Morgan 1996). Exactly the same points can be made about communities. Like families, communities have become far more diverse in terms of their form, as is readily apparent in the proliferation of types of communities that have been identified as being founded not only on commonality of place but also on interests and identities (Crow and Maclean 2006). At the same time, this process of change as a movement away from a standard notion of community nevertheless involves continuity in terms of what the members of these increasingly diverse communities do, and also what they understand themselves to be doing. If communities and families have had to change in order for communities and families to continue to exist, it is a worthwhile exercise to ask just how much has changed. At the very least, reports of the death of the family and of community appear, on the evidence available, to be somewhat premature.

References

Allan, G. and Crow, G. (2001) *Families, Households and Society*, Basingstoke: Palgrave.

Bauman, Z. (2001) *Community: Seeking safety in an insecure world*, Cambridge: Polity.

Beck, U. (1992) *Risk Society: Towards a new modernity*, Cambridge: Polity.

Beck-Gernsheim, E. (2002) *Reinventing the Family: In search of new lifestyles*, Cambridge: Polity.

Bell, C. (1977) 'Reflections on the Banbury re-study', in C. Bell and H. Newby (eds) *Doing Sociological Research*, London: George Allen and Unwin, pp.47–62.

Bell, C. and Newby, H. (1971) *Community Studies: An introduction to the sociology of the local community*, London: George Allen and Unwin.

Bryson, L. and Thompson, F. (1972) *An Australian Newtown: Life and leadership in a working-class suburb*, Melbourne: Penguin.

Bryson, L. and Winter, I. (1999) *Social Change, Suburban Lives: An Australian newtown 1960s to 1990s*, St Leonards, NSW: Allen and Unwin.

Burgoyne, J. and Clark, D. (1984) *Making a go of it: A study of stepfamilies in Sheffield*, London: Routledge and Kegan Paul.

Butler, T. with Robson, G. (2003) *London Calling: The middle classes and the remaking of inner London*, Oxford: Berg.

Cheal, D. (1991) *Family and the State of Theory*, London: Harvester Wheatsheaf.

Cheal, D. (2002) *Sociology of Family Life*, Basingstoke: Palgrave.

Crow, G. (2000) 'Developing sociological arguments through community studies', *International Journal of Social Research Methodology* 3(3): 173–87.

Crow, G. (2002a) 'Community studies: Fifty years of theorization', *Sociological Research Online* 7(3) http://www.socresonline.org.uk/7/3/crow.html

Crow, G. (2002b) *Social Solidarities: Theories, identities and social change*, Buckingham: Open University Press.

Crow, G. (2004) 'People like us, places like ours: developments in urban sociology', *Sociological Review* 52(4): 592–8.

Crow, G. (2005) *The Art of Sociological Argument*, Basingstoke: Palgrave.

Crow, G. and Maclean, C. (2006) 'Community' in G. Payne (ed.) *Social Divisions*, Second edition. Basingstoke: Palgrave.

Davies, C. and Charles, N. (2002) 'The Piano in the Parlour: Methodological issues in the conduct of a restudy', *Sociological Research Online* 7(2) http://www.socresonline.org.uk/7/2/davies.html

Dench, G., Gavron, K. and Young, M. (2006) *The New East End: Kinship, race and conflict*, London: Profile Books.

Finch, J. and Mason, J. (1993) *Negotiating Family Responsibilities*, London: Routledge.

Foster, J. (1999) *Docklands: Cultures in conflict, worlds in collision*, London: UCL Press.

Gershuny, J. (2000) *Changing Times: Work and leisure in postindustrial society*, Oxford: Oxford University Press.

Glucksmann, M. (2000) *Cottons and Casuals: The gendered organization of labour in time and space*, Durham: Sociologypress.

Hareven, T. (2000) *Families, History and Social Change: Life-course and cross-cultural perspectives*, Boulder: Westview.

Holme, A. (1985) *Housing and Young Families in East London*, London: Routledge and Kegan Paul.

Hornsby, A. (1998) 'Surfing the net for community: A Durkheimian analysis of electronic gatherings', in P. Kivisto (ed.) *Illuminating Social Life: Classical and contemporary theory revisited*, Thousand Oaks: Pine Forge Press.

Jamieson, L. (1998) *Intimacy: Personal relationships in modern societies*, Cambridge: Polity.

Keller, S. (2003) *Community: Pursuing the dream, living the reality*, Princeton, NJ: Princeton University Press.

Lassiter, L., Goodall, H., Campbell, E. and Johnson, M. (eds) (2004) *The Other Side of Middletown: Exploring Muncie's African American Community*, Lanham, MD: AltaMira Press.

Lynd, R. and Lynd, H. (1929) *Middletown: A study in contemporary American Culture*, London: Constable.

McRae, S. (1999) 'Introduction: family and household change in Britain', in S. McRae (ed.) *Changing Britain: Families and households in the 1990s*, Oxford: Oxford University Press.

Marris, P. (1987) *Meaning and Action: Community planning and conceptions of change*, London: Routledge and Kegan Paul.

Morgan, D. (1996) *Family Connections: An introduction to family studies*, Cambridge: Polity.

Mumford, K. and Power, A. (2003) *East Enders: Family and community in East London*, Bristol: Policy Press.

Nicolaievsky, B. and Maenchen-Helfen, O. (1976) *Karl Marx: Man and Fighter*, London: Penguin.

Pahl, R. (1984) *Divisions of Labour*, Oxford: Blackwell.

Ribbens McCarthy, J, Edwards, R. and Gillies, V. (2003) *Making Families: Moral tales of parenting and step-parenting*, Durham: Sociologypress.

Roberts, E. (1984) *A Woman's Place: An oral history of working-class women 1890–1940*, Oxford: Blackwell.

Rosser, C. and Harris, C. (1965) *The Family and Social Change: A study of family and kinship in a South Wales town*, London: Routledge and Kegan Paul.

Savage, M., Bagnall, G. and Longhurst, B. (2005) *Globalization and Belonging*, London: Sage.

Scheper-Hughes, N. (2001) *Saints, Scholars and Schizophrenics: Mental illness in rural Ireland*, Berkeley: University of California Press.

Smart, C. and Neale, B. (1999) *Family Fragments?*, Cambridge: Polity.

Stacey, J. (1998) *Brave New Families: Stories of domestic upheaval in late twentieth-century America*, Berkeley: University of California Press.

Stacey, M. (1960) *Tradition and Change: A study of Banbury*, Oxford: Oxford University Press.

Stacey, M., Batstone, E., Bell, C. and Murcott, A. (1975) *Power, Persistence and Change: A second study of Banbury*, London: Routledge and Kegan Paul.

Stein, M. (1964) *The Eclipse of Community: An interpretation of American studies*, New York: Harper and Row.

Warwick, D. and Littlejohn, G. (1992) *Coal, Capital and Culture: A Sociological Analysis of Mining Communities in West Yorkshire*, London:Routledge.

Williams, W. M. (1963) *A West Country Village: Ashworthy*, London: Routledge and Kegan Paul.

Young, M. (1988) *The Metronomic Society: Natural rhythms and human timetables*, London: Thames and Hudson.

Young, M. and Willmott, P. (1957) *Family and Kinship in East London*, London: Routledge and Kegan Paul.

Young, M. and Willmott, P. (1975) *The Symmetrical Family: A study of work and leisure in the London region*, Harmondsworth: Penguin.

Chapter 3

Are community studies still 'good to think with'?

David H. J. Morgan

Introduction

There are numerous ways of defining or approaching the idea of 'community' and a common move in writings on the subject is to list these diverse definitions. (For some of these definitions and guides to recent discussions see Bauman 2001; Crow and Allan 1994; Delanty 2003). It is perhaps slightly easier to identify some of the core concerns linked with the study of community: boundaries, belonging and identity, inter-connectedness, density, embeddedness, and so on. These concerns, with different emphases, reoccur within the more extended discussions.

An alternative, overlapping strategy is to indicate some of the different ways in which the word 'community' functions and, at the outset, I list four possible complex usages:

1   As a key idea or a master narrative in sociological analysis. Nisbet, for example, sees 'community' as one of five key ideas within the sociological tradition and as probably the most important of these (Nisbet 1996/1966). In this context, 'community' may be seen, for example, at the end of a continuum or in opposition to societies or social organisations dominated by principles of rationality and the market economy.
2   As a sense of 'we-ness', identity, difference, and belonging. Specifically identified 'communities' are indicated here and there may be discussions about whether a particular location may justifiably be described as a community. For example, Gans asked this question in relation to the new housing development 'Levittown', and came to the conclusion that as a whole it could not be so defined (Gans 1967).
3   As an ideological or rhetorical device stating who 'we' are and, perhaps more importantly, who we are not. Recent debates about Britishness or Englishness may use this rhetoric of community.
4   As 'community' studies, representing a particular approach to sociological analysis.

My central concern in this chapter is with this last understanding, although these other themes also appear. I am dealing primarily with a cluster (or several clusters) of studies conducted mainly within the British Isles and identified by, among others, Cohen, Crow and Allan, and Frankenberg (Cohen 1985, 1982, 1986; Crow and Allan 1994; Frankenberg, 1966. See also Edwards *et al.* 2005). Several of these studies have reached the status of canonical texts within British sociology and continue to be found on numerous student reading lists. I shall not attempt to summarise these studies or to draw out their key features. Rather, I am concerned with what we may continue to get out of these studies and how they may continue to contribute to the wider practices of thinking sociologically. I am also concerned with the possible importance of these studies once we stray beyond the more territorial understanding of 'community', which might be seen as an implicit feature of these studies.

Part of my interest in these studies comes from my intellectual autobiography. Studies of Bethnal Green, Welsh villages, a Cumbrian farming community, and a Yorkshire mining village were among my first introductions to sociology and I have returned to them, in all kinds of different ways, from time to time ever since my undergraduate days. I find this is true for several other sociologists of my generation and later ones.

Partly, also, my interest is in community studies as a methodology or particular approach to sociological analysis (Brunt 2001). Whatever particular techniques are used, a key element involves some degree of extended familiarity with the location under investigation and some degree of sharing in the (working and/or residential) lives of the inhabitants. This kind of approach has several further consequences. These include a link, explicit or implicit, between personal biography and social analysis, some kind of holistic understanding, and the development of what Geertz calls 'thick description' (Geertz 1973).

My title, as most readers will recognise, derives from Levi-Strauss's analysis of totemism, in which he argues that particular animals and plants are chosen as totemic objects not because they are good to eat but because they are good to think with (Levi-Strauss 1963). I see community studies not simply as sources of information about particular locations (the equivalent of being 'good to eat') but because they can still raise questions and provide insight into the heart of sociological analysis. I hope to be able to demonstrate that they are still good to think with despite, in some cases, their relative antiquity.

A North Wales Village

I shall begin to develop my arguments through the use of an extended case. For this I have chosen *A North Wales Village* by Isabel Emmett, published in 1964. I have chosen this example for a variety of reasons. First, it is part of my biography. Emmett was one of the first persons I met when I went to Manchester, and during the subsequent years I gained much from her socio-logical imagination and high intellectual standards. Her book was published shortly after we had arrived at Manchester to work on a factory study, under the direct supervision of Ronnie Frankenberg and Valdo Pons, with Max Gluckman as the senior investigator. Second, I think that the study was somewhat overshadowed by some of the more canonical studies within British community studies; her work only receives a passing men-tion, for example, in Crow and Allan's survey (Crow and Allan 1994). Third, I think that the study has considerable, subtle richness and serves as a good source of themes to illustrate my present concerns.

Emmett's fieldwork was carried out between 1958 and 1962. The partic-ular locality, which she calls 'Llan', was selected for the simplest of reasons: she was married to a native of the parish. It is also important to note that she was English and not a Welsh speaker. This awareness of difference informs much of her analysis, as it informs several other similar studies. She argues briefly, but cogently, that information cannot be separated from interpretation and she sees her task as making seemingly strange or irra-tional behaviour comprehensible. She thus locates herself in the tradition clearly represented by Evans-Pritchard and his analysis of Azande witch-craft (Evans-Pritchard 1937). Emmett seeks to avoid psychological explanations of behaviour, seeking instead an understanding of that behav-iour in the context of the community within which it takes place. This thoroughly sociological understanding of her project, looking outward from the particular community to wider issues, makes the study especially appropriate for my purposes.

Emmett's analytical strategy is to focus on three paradoxes:

1   There was a relative absence of class distinctions within the immediate community itself despite the fact that Llan was part of a wider class society.
2   A large amount of salmon poaching took place within the area despite the fact that the fish were hardly ever sold and did not form a signifi-cant part of the local diet.
3   There were, at the time of research, relatively high rates of illegitimacy (and other indices of premarital sexual behaviour) despite the fact that the teachings of the chapel were an influential force in the community.

Linking these apparent paradoxes is her analysis of the overriding impor-tance of a sense of Welshness.

I shall develop the second two paradoxes a little further. Poaching salmon is economically unimportant. It may be an exciting activity but, again, this is not the central concern. The poachers, she argues, deploying their knowledge, skill, and use of local grapevines in order to defeat the river bailiff (who represents English interests), are 'partisans in peacetime'. Poaching is only one of a range of practices which serve to maintain a sense of Welsh identity.

Turning to the third paradox, it might be possible to see the relatively high rates of illegitimacy as a sign of the weakening role of the chapel. However, as long ago as 1847 (a time of intense religious fervour), Reverend J. W. Trevor is quoted as stating that '… fornication is not regarded as a vice, scarcely as a frailty, by the common people in Wales' (Emmett 1964: 102–3). This continuing divergence between teaching and practice was also found in the women known (at least to some of the men) as 'good things'. These women were not prostitutes but were seen, to use more modern terminology, as 'easy lays'. No particular stigma seemed to attach itself to this identity or to the actual practices. Here, as in all communities one might suppose, there was a flexible interpretation of the dominant moral code represented by the chapel.

Again, Emmett links this to the theme of Welshness, saying that 'Welshness is the primary value; deacon and drunkard are friends, old schisms become unimportant' (ibid. 13). This analysis, linking apparent paradoxes with issues to do with Welsh identity, is also connected with her insightful discussion of the role of 'not-knowing' in the local community. This has many layers of meaning. Not knowing, or claiming not to know, may be a way of living alongside your neighbours in a relatively close community. It reflects, further, an understanding that knowledge is a form of currency which must be carefully guarded and only given out or exchanged in small portions. This contrasts with the English visitors who, perhaps over-eager to integrate into the locality, squander their knowledge at the first opportunity. Hence 'not knowing' is yet another weapon in the armoury of the peacetime partisans.

I hope that this short account has given something of the flavour of Emmett's analysis and has made a case for its continuing relevance. It clearly tells the reader something about a small part of North Wales at a particular point of time but that is not its main relevance. My interest is in the study's particular insights and analytical strategies, and how the relevance of these might even be greater today. For example, the study has a lot to tell us about the process of building and maintaining boundaries – an important theme in the analysis of communities – and thus provides a link between earlier studies and some of the more recent studies which focus more explicitly on these issues (Cohen 1982, 1986). Here we might also see insights into the experiences and practices of colonialism, as well as the responses to colonialism.

Another area of continuing significance is the study of everyday or practical moralities (as opposed to the more formal, and often prescriptive, analysis practised by philosophers or parsons). A more sociological understanding of morality recognises that people are often faced with multiple, and sometimes conflicting, obligations and moral choices and that, at this more everyday level, involve decisions and negotiations. Thus we can link the everyday accommodations and tacit agreements within a community such as Llan to more recent discussions of the making of moral decisions within family settings (Finch and Mason 1993; Ribbens McCarthy *et al.* 2003; Smart and Neale 1999).

Perhaps most of all, *A North Wales Village* contributes to an understanding of community in terms of language and stories. This is not simply a question of the Welsh language versus the English language, but of the richness of local references and naming practices. Emmett writes:

> This history is not one of important events: the two world wars left the lives of most Llan people unmarked. It is a history of scandal and jokes, a gossip history, whose power on people and beauty for people is hard to express. Part of the power derives from the fact that everyone is familiar with that past; anyone can describe it.
>
> (Emmett 1964: 10)

Another way of describing community, perhaps, is in terms of a nexus of stories (Morgan 2005). I shall return to this theme.

Thinking with and through community studies

I chose Emmett's *A North Wales Village* to open up some of the more general themes that I wish to discuss. I could have chosen any one of a couple of dozen or more such studies; all of them, in different ways and with different emphases, move between the general and the particular, raising issues to do with the place of locally lived lives within wider divisions or movements of social change. From *Coal Is Our Life* (Dennis *et al.* 1969) for example, I might gain insights into issues of class and gender, just as from *Village on the Border* (Frankenberg 1957) I gain illumination into political processes.

There is little doubt that the local and immediate can still fascinate the reader and that community studies may provide information about and insights into worlds which we have lost or which we seem about to lose. Some of this may reflect nostalgia and may be linked to the continuing popularity of community-based soap operas. But it is also clear that some of the earlier studies now form, when properly interrogated, part of the body of resources open to social historians. *Family and Kinship in East London* (Young and Willmott 1957), one of the first studies I read as an undergraduate, is now 50 years old. The process by which yesterday's sociology becomes today's history is perhaps one of the less heralded and discussed relationships between the two disciplines.

However, as I hope will have been made clear, my argument is less to do with the information that community studies might provide and more to do with the ways in which they encourage reflection and theorising. Although it is perhaps less apparent in Emmett's study, one such area is to do with the process of stability and change. This everyday contrast frequently appears in the community studies I am concerned with and forms the basis of Frankenberg's overview of this body of work (Frankenberg 1966; Morgan 2005). At the very least, community studies may encourage a degree of caution in the face of grand narratives of historical change such as, for example, those couched in terms such as 'individualisation' or 'globalisation'.

Clearly a methodology which focuses upon the particular and upon locally embedded meanings will tend to be, at best, sceptical about theories which operate at a more macro level. This is not to say that community studies were unable to handle social change. Indeed structural economic and social change was not far from many of the classic British accounts – Frankenberg's *Village on the Border* is a prominent example (1957). But the community studies approach encourages us to see these processes from the more immediate level of experience and meaning rather than from the perspective of models which pay little attention to the local. Put another way, it is the direction of analysis with which we are concerned. Rather than seeing particular communities as simply illustrating more generalised social processes, the particular studies can be used to elaborate wider analytical themes.

This argument has several different, although related, strands. First, community studies remind us of the persistence of cultural diversity within the boundaries of a single modern state. (It is worth remembering that most of the community studies with which I am concerned were conducted well before more recent debates about 'multiculturalism'.) This theme of diversity is one stressed by Cohen (1982; 1986) as well as works written or edited by Frankenberg. Cohen refers to a 'marvellous complexity' (1982: 2) and the importance of an 'ethnography of locality' – a term which might well be developed in place of the older term 'community studies'. We have no reason to suppose that such diversity and complexity has in any way diminished. Indeed it might have increased. Where there has been change it is in terms of the nature of such diversity and complexity.

Such studies, however, do not simply demonstrate the continuing existence of cultural diversity within the British Isles. They also demonstrate how a 'sense of difference' is constructed and maintained. In other words, they are concerned with one of the most fundamental social processes and a core concern of sociology: the construction and maintenance of boundaries and identities. Such boundaries are rarely physical or administrative (although they may be coterminous with these), but are symbolic boundaries. They may be given through history and location but they require considerable ongoing work, individual and collective, to reaffirm them. This work may include use of language and telling of stories, participation in rituals, preparation and enjoyment of food, and mobilisation of others in support of some cause. The awareness of difference and of one's own culture occurs, as Cohen puts it, 'when they stand at its boundaries' (Cohen 1982: 3). Such awareness defines who we are and who they are and, equally, who I am and who you are.

This work does not deny that any particular community might not be divided or more complex than a simple 'we' claim might suggest. To quote Cohen again: 'To put it another way, the boundary as the community's public face is symbolically simple; but, as the object of internal discourse, it is symbolically complex' (Cohen 1986: 13). Indeed, it could be argued that part of this 'we' sense is a recognition of such internal complexities that are not accessible to outsiders. One of the roles of the observer, therefore, is to mediate between the simple models suggested by the public appearance and the more complex reality experienced on a day to day basis by the local participants.

This mediation is clear, for example, in Whyte's *Street Corner Society* where the contrast is between the rather negative public image of a dysfunctional urban neighbourhood and the daily complexities and subtle differentiations that take place within the area (Whyte 1955). Damer, achieves something similar in his discussion of Glasgow's 'wine alley' (Damer 1989). Turning back to Emmett's study, at a superficial level there might appear to be a straightforward barrier between Welsh and English that is manifested in numerous daily encounters and more generalised representations. Internally, however, we see a complex nexus of stories and shifting local divisions and identities in which even the English can appear as complex individuals. Such boundary work is, I argue, a fundamental social process and one not likely to be suspended in the face of individualisation or globalisation. Paradoxically, in looking at the ways in which people differentiate themselves and assert their specialness, they are also announcing what they share with members of other similarly bounded communities.

The drawing, maintaining, and possible modification of symbolic boundaries is a fundamental social process that is not simply confined to locally defined communities. We find similar discussions in, for example, the sociologies of race relations, religion, and nationalism. But even in these more general, perhaps even global, issues we may still discover that the more locally based analysis can illuminate the more general processes. A study of a single parish could illuminate our understanding of Catholicism just as a study of something like the Notting Hill carnival could have something to say about more general issues of race and ethnicity.

This movement back and forth between the general and the particular is one of the reasons why community studies have an abiding value. It is, for example, no accident that so many community studies (especially those more clearly located in a social anthropological tradition) are concerned with gossip. Gossip, as a form of exchange and sharing, creates and recreates personal ties and community identities. To be a recipient of gossip is to receive some recognition as a co-participant in a particular set of relations and to incur an obligation to share gossip in the future. Even the expressed disapproval of gossip may become part of these processes of acknowledging and recognising ties and membership.

One particular and striking example of the links that can be made between apparently disparate settings is provided by Frankenberg. In his analysis of 'taking the blame and passing the buck', he argues that the processes within a wartime Cabinet committee could be illuminated from his study of a football committee in his *Village on the Border* (Frankenberg 1957; 1972). Although everyday conflicts and divisions in war and peace, and in work and leisure, are frequently explained in terms of individual personalities, this kind of social anthropological approach can demonstrate the incompleteness of such accounts, however popular and widespread they might be. As with the case of gossip, there are more fundamental social processes at work.

An important area where it is possible to explore this interplay between the general and the particular in the context of community studies is in the area of gender and sexuality. Community studies, unlike some of the earlier studies of work and the workplace, were always aware that such locations included both men and women and that gender was an important social division within them. Gender was, for example, very much at the fore in one of the most widely quoted British community studies, *Coal Is Our Life* (Dennis *et al.* 1969), and represents a key division in Frankenberg's study (1957). In the case of the former study, a dominant theme was the difference, the sharp contrast, between the mine and the home. This difference was practically and symbolically mapped on to the differences between men and women. Gender differences and the difference between home and work reinforced each other and pervaded other areas of community life, especially leisure.

Issues of sexuality were, perhaps unusually, not ignored in this account. One of the most memorable passages deals with a queue outside a cinema that was showing the Marilyn Monroe film, *Niagara*. The men were speculating on what they would like to do with the star of the movie while the women were mocking the men's pretensions. They were casting ribald doubts on the men's ability to satisfy Marilyn Monroe and demonstrating some clear signs of sexual antagonism. Had there been some women on the research team it is possible that further signs of heterosexual tension might have been discovered.

It could be argued that the researchers here were drawing upon fairly unproblematic notions of sexual divisions, differences between men and women, without exploring in any great depth the nature of sexual divisions within capitalism. While sexual divisions were explored in some detail here, it is probably true to say that the main social divisions with which they were concerned were those of class. We have to wait a decade or so before we begin to see more theoretical explorations of the relationships between class and gender or between capitalism and patriarchy. Similarly, it can be argued that, in this and several other community studies of the time, gender was a matter of the difference between men and women, not the relationships between women and between men. However, it is often possible to re-read such studies in order to rediscover themes of, say, masculinity (Morgan 1992).

With the development of feminist scholarship and practice we begin to get a greater awareness of the importance of gender not only in community studies, but also in increasingly wide areas of sociological enquiry. Gender came to be seen as much more pervasive and much more complex. The sexual division of labour was to do with divisions in employment, in the home, and with the relationships between these two sites. Further, a political or ethical dimension was introduced; the relationships between men and women were not only ones of difference but also of exploitation and oppression.

As the growth of more gender-aware studies of communities, workplaces, leisure activities, and so on continued, we also began to see another shift of emphasis. The community or the workplace was not simply an arena where gender divisions were played out according to some pre-existing script, but they were also places where people enacted or *did* gender rather than simply being the carriers of gendered identities. Further, the workplace and the community were also sites where people *did* sexuality as a set of practices as well as doing gender.

A striking illustration of this approach is found in Linda McDowell's study of the City of London (McDowell 1997). This is an example of a working environment which also has some strong community-like features, including overlaps between work and leisure, networks linking different workplaces, and a clear sense of identity and symbolic place. While the City has undergone considerable change it still retains some of these community-like features. The emphasis on the need for new recruits to 'fit in' suggests some features of an ongoing community-like culture. Gender and sexuality are key themes in McDowell's analysis and are not simply questions of divisions of labour or, in particular, the extent to which women have been recruited for key City positions and institutions. The analysis is also about the extent to which gender and sexuality come to be seen as key themes in shaping the culture of the organisations and working environments. Hence there are accounts of the ways in which women are 'marked' as women within these working environments, with a particular emphasis upon embodied appearance and dress. Similarly the dominant language of the City reflects masculine concerns of war, sport, and heterosexuality. In one illuminating phrase, McDowell writes that 'The young men in corporate finance presented an astonishingly physical uniform appearance ...' (McDowell 1997: 187). Gender and sexuality are, therefore, not simply 'added on' to a study of a working environment but are central to a full understanding of the community-like features of that environment.

Over the past few decades, therefore, it is possible to see a set of exchanges in the development of community studies and the theorising of gender and sexuality. Some of the earlier community studies provided valuable source material for the exploration of gender divisions as the study of such divisions became more prominent within sociological enquiry. Later developments in the theorising of gender and sexuality – including feminist, performative, postmodern approaches – came to inform community studies or studies of the workplace. Community studies, both past and more recent, continue to be a valuable source, not simply of data or information, but of ideas and understanding about how gender works in the conduct of everyday lives. Community studies aid in the development of gendered thinking.

Beyond the local

In looking at a study like McDowell's study of the City of London we are moving away from what many people might understand by the term 'community', with its strong identification with a locality where there is considerable overlap between home and work. The people in this particular study, and similar ones, work in this environment and associate with each other out of working hours, but probably live in a wide variety of locations. However, a major theme in the analysis of community (and one stressed in the earlier commentary by Nisbet) is that the idea of community is not to be confined to local studies of villages or areas within cities which have clear and largely recognised boundaries. To use a well-established sociological distinction, 'cosmopolitans' may belong to communities as much as 'locals'.

In the course of his studies, Frankenberg comes to prefer the approach outlined by Max Gluckman: '... a lot of people co-operating and disputing within the limits of an established system of relations and cultures' (Frankenberg 1982: 5; Gluckman 1958: 35). There is an openness, perhaps even vagueness, about this definition. What, for example, is a 'lot' of people? Yet it removes the idea of community from particular locations on a map and points to the systemic connections between relations and cultures. Further, it provides a clear corrective to any nostalgic visions of harmonious communities; conflict, dispute, and division are as much at the heart of community life as are cooperation and mutual support. Such conflicts and divisions are clearly identifiable in the studies by Frankenberg, Emmett, Dennis, Henriques and Slaughter, and McDowell, among others, that are referred to in these pages. Further, such recognition of the fact of conflict does not exclude the possibilities of community identities and the drawing of community boundaries.

There are certain communities, especially those based upon religious or ethnic identities, which have both a local and a national, or even global, referent. As has already been mentioned, it is possible to explore more general issues of religious practice or ethnic identity through the study of a locality or a locally based place of worship. Hannerz's study of *Soulside* considers the extent to which such locally based anthropological studies can contribute to a more general understanding of racial tension within the United

States as a whole (Hannerz 1969). Within Britain, there have been studies of local Pakistani communities which are clearly not just about particular areas of Rochdale or Manchester (Anwar 1985; Werbner 1990). Further, such studies do not simply illuminate what might frequently be identified as 'social problems', but also contribute to our understanding of wider socio-logical problems as well such as the interplays between class, ethnicity, and gender or the mobilisation of informal support through social networks.

I select a religious study which is not usually understood to be a com-munity study: *When Prophecy Fails* (Festinger *et al.* 1956). As a full-blown community study it is probably deficient in several ways and we would need to know a lot more about the locality and how the people earn a living and conduct their everyday lives. Nevertheless, it is a locally based study of a cult predicting the end of the world and what happens when the prophesy fails to come about. The 'community' is not so much the locality, of Lake City, but a small and fluid network of believers who have a shared back-ground in various esoteric cults and movements. The authors, social psychologists, deploy and develop their theories of cognitive dissonance through the use of this particular case study. Despite the authors' more gen-eral theoretical interest, we never quite lose the sense of the more immediate concerns and issues. True to our understanding of the idea of community, there are accounts of differences and conflicts as well as of the boundaries which are established around this cult.

There will always be some debate about the extent to which local studies of particular religious or ethnic communities can illuminate the whole of which they form a part. However, there can be little doubt that they can provide such illumination as well as making contributions to wider processes of social theorising. But it is equally obvious that a study of, say, a particular Catholic parish will leave out a lot if the reader wishes to obtain a fuller understanding of that particular faith. Particular religious commu-nities, such as a parish, are related to other communities within the same faith in at least two ways. First, and perhaps more rhetorically, there may be some reference to the worldwide Catholic community or some similar des-ignation. It is doubtful whether the conventional methods of community studies can capture this particular discursive understanding, although the numerous and extensive debates about the meaning of community (espe-cially around themes of boundary drawing and identity) might provide some illumination. The worldwide and varied response to the death of a Pope might provide the basis of an extensive case study of this particular understanding of community.

Second, however, we may refer to the Catholic Church as a global organ-isation and we may be interested, for example, in the ways in which men at the upper levels of the hierarchy, such as bishops, cardinals, or senior schol-ars, might themselves be seen as a community. Certainly, Gluckman's relatively open definition could readily be applied here and could become the basis of, say, a study of the processes of electing a new Pope. In any event, it would seem to be a reasonable assumption that a group of people at the top of any (religious, cultural, economic, or political) hierarchy will come to cooperate and dispute; these exchanges may happen on a face-to-face basis in conferences or conclaves, or perhaps increasingly through email and the mass media.

An example of this sense of community (referring to communities of interests, practices, and knowledge) is provided by the anthropologist Ulf Hannerz in his discussion of urban anthropology:

> Obviously by now [1980] urban anthropologists are forming a community. They apply for their own specialist slots in anthropology departments, they meet in their own conferences, and they write in no small part for each other when they do not write textbooks to teach students about cities.
>
> (Hannerz 1980: 2)

It is likely that most readers of this chapter will have experienced something of this sense of community; it is also probable that few of them would feel any hesitation in using this word to describe their involvement in similar academic or professional circles. To quote Hannerz again: 'As Gans puts it, everyone might not know everyone else, but they know something about everyone else' (ibid. 5). Or, one might add, they know how to find out about anyone else within this particular defined community.

Such interest communities, often global in scope, can easily be brought within the ambit of community studies and understanding them can be aided by a reading of some of the older examples of this craft. There are two further areas which deserve attention. The first is the growth of 'virtual communities' and, equally, of scholarly attention to these sets of practices. An example of a virtual community might be provided by the website *Eons.com,* which is for baby boomers (and older) only: '"Social-networking sites are wonderful for people of my generation," says Bloom who lives in Maryland. "We've always been really social, and they're all about developing a community"' (Vencat 2007: 36).

Virtual communities would seem to have much in common with ideas about postmodernity as they are often 'polymorphous, highly personalized and often expressive' (Delanty 2003: 166). Yet, as Delanty also points out, such virtual communities may be associated with more 'traditional' forms, such as extended families. Further virtual communities may be associated with, or contribute to the development of, actual social events and interactions.

The overall significance of virtual communities for, among other things, understandings of community, senses of embodiment, and ideas of democracy remains a matter for considerable controversy (Holmes 1997). For example, are they a significant response to the supposed loss of community within society or part of the problem, since at their core is an individual in front of a screen (Willson 1997)? Does it matter that individuals participating in a virtual community may disguise all kinds of details about themselves, including gender, ethnicity, and age? And is it the case that, despite the constant use of the language of space, 'networks do not reproduce space, they eliminate it' (Chesher 1997: 83)? And, if so, does that matter for the analysis of community, given that we have already released the idea of community from any spatial anchorage? At this point it might be prudent to see some significance in the fact that participants frequently use the word 'community' to describe their practices and to see this as a starting point for further analysis.

The second development which needs to be considered has to do with the idea of 'personal communities', which is frequently associated with social network analysis. Wellman defines these communities as 'intimate and active ties with friends, neighbours and work mates as well as kin' (Wellman 1990: 195, quoted in Pahl and Spencer 2004: 74). Here the focus is upon an individual's role in the active creation of communities (which may also take on lives of their own) and a notion of community where the notion of locality and shared space, if not entirely absent, is severely limited. Such communities are ego-centred, which means that it is unlikely that a member of someone's personal community network will have a completely coterminus personal network. Nevertheless, these networks may also be significant in the mobilisation of social support and social capital (Phillipson et al. 2004). Following Gluckman's definition, they may also be a location for social disputes (although this is perhaps less explored than the more positive features). Further, there is no reason why there might not be some overlap between personal communities and virtual communities (although, again, this is probably less explored).

There are, therefore, all kinds of ways in which community studies may take us beyond the immediate locality, moving from a particularly identified community (as on a map) to communities based upon interests and knowledge on the internet or in personal networks. Further, our understanding of community must increasingly take into account the multiple communities of which an individual might be a part: 'Organized more like a network, community today is abstract and lacks visibility and unity, and as a result is more an imagined condition than a symbolically shaped reality based on fixed reference points' (Delanty 2003: 188). The community (or communities) of choice parallel (and may be closely linked to) the 'families of choice' that can be seen as a feature of modern intimate life.

Conclusion

Some communities of interest, virtual communities, and personal communities may seem a long way from the villages and clearly bounded locations that were at the heart of British community studies and which frequently appeared on the titles of monographs. Nevertheless, these studies (and studies which continue, to some measure, within this tradition) did not simply record worlds we have lost, but remain good frameworks for thinking. This is because the method, which allows themes to develop in the course of the analysis and seeks to explore some sense of the whole, is still an important feature of sociological enquiry. Good community studies, whenever or wherever they are conducted, allow for some sense of interplay between historical change and immediately located experiences, between the local and the national or the global, and between the particular and the general. For example, Frankenberg's 'morphological continuum', developed in his overview of *Communities in Britain* (1966), contains a whole range of theoretical ideas and methodological tools. Many of these ideas and tools focus on social networks and their structure and functioning. Whether such a continuum could be extended to include personal communities and virtual communities is a matter for debate, but it is certain that some of the ideas developed here, and in the community studies tradition in general, are of continuing relevance.

Much, of course, depends upon the ways in which community studies are read. They can be read for information about particular locations in the past or as examples of a particular body of work, author, or school. But I suspect that community studies will be read actively, engaging the reader's own experiences and personal understandings of community. At times the reader might think 'how different!' and at other times 'how much the same!'. Whatever the response, it is likely that this active reading will be part of a process of thinking through community studies to the continuing ideas and practices of community.

I want to conclude with my idea of community as a nexus of stories. This is not the only way to think about the community but it is an additional way which might have something to contribute. In many communities, whether local, based on shared interests, or personal networks, part of the everyday currency is the telling of stories. They are a source of pleasure, local knowledge and information, and possibly moral instruction. Stories also contribute to a sense of personal identity and connectedness, although they may also reflect, or be a source of, divisions and disputes. As Emmett and many other observers of community life have shown, stories are of particular relevance in particular localities where they may go back several generations. But stories are also part of the way in which members of interest- or knowledge-based communities relate to each other and, I should suggest, are part of the way in which personal communities work. Stories may also have their part in virtual communities, although perhaps in this instance it is more a question of shared points of reference and uses of language. Stories remain an important way in which individuals understand their worlds and locate themselves within them. The stories that ethnographers tell, perhaps at some removed stage, may also have a part to play.

References

Anwar, M. (1985) *Pakistanis in Britain: A Sociological Study*, London: New Century.

Bauman, Z. (2001) *Community: Seeking Safety in an Insecure World*, Cambridge: Polity.

Brunt, L. (2001) 'Into the community', in P. Atkinson, A. Coffey, S. Delamont, J. Lofland and L. Lofland (eds) *Handbook of Ethnography*, London: Sage.

Chesher, C. (1997) 'The ontology of digital domains', in D. Holmes (ed.) *Virtual Politics: Identity and Community in Cyberspace*, London: Sage.

Cohen, A.P. (1985) *The Symbolic Construction of Community*, London: Tavistock.

Cohen, A.P. (ed.) (1982) *Belonging: Identity and Social Organisation in British Rural Communities*, Manchester: MUP.

Cohen, A.P. (ed.) (1986) *Symbolising Boundaries: Identity and Diversity in British Cultures*, Manchester: MUP.

Crow, G. and Allan, G. (1994) *Community Life: An Introduction to Local Social Relations*, London: Harvester/Wheatsheaf.

Damer, S. (1989) *From Moorepark to 'Wine Alley': The Rise and Fall of a Glasgow Housing Scheme*, Edinburgh: Edinburgh University Press.

Delanty, G. (2003) *Community*, London: Routledge.

Dennis, N., Henriques, F. and Slaughter, C. (1969) *Coal Is Our Life: An Analysis of a Yorkshire Mining Community*, London: Tavistock.

Edwards, J., Macdonald, S. and Savage, M. (eds) (2005) 'Community, continuity and change in the study of Britain: A Festschrift for Ronnie Frankenberg', Special issue, *The Sociological Review*, 53(4).

Emmett, I. (1964) *A North Wales Village: A Social Anthropological Study*, London: Routledge & Kegan Paul.

Evans-Pritchard, E. E. (1937) *Witchcraft, Oracles and Magic Among the Azande*, Oxford: Clarendon Press.

Festinger, L., Riecken, H. W. and Schachter, S. (1956) *When Prophecy Fails*, Minneapolis: University of Minnesota Press.

Finch, J. and Mason, J. (1993) *Negotiating Family Responsibilities*, London: Routledge.

Frankenberg, R. (1957) *Village on The Border*, London: Cohen & West.

Frankenberg, R. (1966) *Communities in Britain: Social Life in Town and Country*, Harmondsworth: Penguin.

Frankenberg, R. (1972) 'Taking the blame and passing the buck, or, the carpet of Agamemnon: an essay on the problems of responsibility, legitimation and triviality' in M. Gluckman (ed.) *The Allocation of Responsibility*, Manchester: MUP.

Frankenberg, R. (ed.) (1982) *Custom and Conflict in British Society*, Manchester: MUP.

Gans, H. J. (1967) *The Levittowners: Anatomy of Suburbia: The Birth of Society and Politics in a New American Town*, London: Allen Lane.

Geertz, C. (1973) *The Interpretation of Cultures*, New York: Basic Books.

Gluckman, M. (1958) *Analysis of a Social Situation in Modern Zululand*, Manchester: MUP.

Hannerz, U. (1969) *Soulside*, New York: Columbia University Press.

Hannerz, U. (1980) *Exploring the City: Inquiries Toward an Urban Anthropology*, New York: Columbia University Press.

Holmes, D. (ed.) (1997) *Virtual Politics: Identity and Community in Cyberspace*, London: Sage.

Levi-Strauss, C. (1963) *Totemism*, Boston, Mass.: Beacon.

McDowell, L. (1997) *Capital Culture: Gender at Work in the City*, Oxford: Blackwell.

Morgan, D. (1992) *Discovering Men*, London: Routledge.

Morgan, D. H. J. (2005) 'Revisiting "Communities in Britain"', *The Sociological Review* 53(4): 641–57.

Nisbet, R.A. (1996/1966) *The Sociological Tradition*, New Brunswick: Transaction Books.

Pahl, R. and Spencer, R. (2004) 'Capturing personal communities', in C. Phillipson, G. Allan and D. Morgan (eds) *Social Networks and Social Exclusion: Sociological and Policy Perspectives*, Aldershot: Ashgate (pp.72–96).

Phillipson, C., Allan, G. and Morgan, D. (eds) (2004) *Social Networks and Social Exclusion: Sociological and Policy Perspectives*, Aldershot: Ashgate.

Ribbens McCarthy, J., Edwards, R. and Gillies, V. (2003) *Making Families: Moral Tales of Parenting and Step-Parenting*, Durham: Sociologypress.

Smart, C. and Neale, B. (1999) *Family Fragments?*, Cambridge: Polity Press.

Vencat, E. F. (2007) 'Netting old friends', *Newsweek*, 5 January: 36–7.

Wellman, B. (1990) 'The place of kinfolk in personal community settings', in DG Unger (ed.) *Families in Community Settings: Interdisciplinary Settings*, New York: Haworth Press.

Werbner, P. (1990) *The Migration Process: Capital, Gifts and Offerings among British Pakistanis*, Oxford: Berg.

Whyte, W. F. (1955) *Street Corner Society: The Social Structure of an Italian Slum*, Chicago: University of Chicago Press.

Willson, M. (1997) 'Community in the abstract: a political and ethical dilemma?', in D. Holmes (ed.) *Virtual politics: Identity and Community in Cyberspace*, London: Sage.

Young, M. and Willmott, P. (1957) *Family and Kinship in East London*, London: Routledge & Kegan Paul.

Chapter 4

Rewriting sexuality and history

Jeffrey Weeks

Living history

We are living in the midst of a long, unfinished but profound revolution that has transformed sexual and intimate life. Since 1945 there have been dramatic changes in family and marriage, erotic behaviour, sexual identities, parenting, relationships between men and women, men and men, women and women, adults and young people, as well as in laws, norms, and values. These changes have remade everyday life in Britain, and in many other parts of the world. But these changes have become so assimilated that the true nature of the transformations is forgotten. They are taken for granted, and the complex history that produced them can all too easily be obliterated. A good index of this is the ways in which the dramatic sex reforms in the second half of the Blair government have been almost completely ignored in discussions of the former Prime Minister's legacy (Weeks 2007: 192). Yet these changes have enshrined the most significant change in the legal framework of sexuality for a hundred years, instituting a new discourse of equality between heterosexuality and homosexuality in the regulation of sexuality. That, in turn, is a response to transformations in the ways in which sexuality and intimacy is lived.

Such is the central argument of my book, *The World We Have Won* (Weeks 2007), and this chapter is, in part, a reflection on the intention and approach of that book. This chapter not only reflects on the book's arguments, but also on the importance I see of relating the present to the past in a constant move between a historic present and a living past. The book focuses on the 'remaking of erotic and intimate life', as the subtitle suggests, since 1945. I take that date as the notional starting point for a variety of reasons: it saw the end of the Second World War and the birth of welfare systems as we still know them; it was the nodal point of the baby boom generation who were so influential in all that happened thereafter; and it happens to be the year of my birth. The last point may be less historically significant than the first two, but it happens to be important to me. More than that, the year forces a form of reflexivity in which the author as historian and sociologist, observer and involved sexual citizen can bear witness to the transformations, deploying his own lived experience as a form of evidence: not as embodied truth, but as one fragment of many truths, a modest contribution to the shaping of a plausible narrative and analysis of the world we have won.

The book's title refers, of course, to Peter Laslett's famous book, *The World We Have Lost* (1965), which helped revolutionise our understanding of the English pre-industrial history of individualism and family life. Laslett was interested in recreating a world that we were ignorant of, and in laying bare the impact of industrialisation on family and domestic life. It is the world created by the industrial revolution that is now disappearing. Paradoxically it is the loss of that world, which displaced the 'world we have lost', which now produces the most passionate nostalgia for a more settled and ordered moral culture than we apparently have today. On the one hand we are offered a vision of a past of tradition, authority, sexual restraint, family discipline, neighbourliness, and good behaviour, where youthful unruliness could easily be curbed by a good clip over the ears by the local bobby. On the other hand, this is counter-posed to the apparent amoral uncertainty or even, according to taste and moral urgency, the chaos of today, where families disintegrate, marriage is in apparently fatal decline, youth is more or less feral, 'anything goes' sexually, perversity is normalised, and 'respect' has all but disappeared (Phillips 1999; Davies 2006).

This latter, morally conservative critique has had a powerful purchase, despite its highly tendentious use of evidence, and underpins the report of the Conservative policy group on social justice led by Duncan Smith (2007), which was widely supported not only in the Tory press (for a critical assessment see Toynbee 2007). Echoes of the position can be traced even amongst leading radical scholars. For example, Zygmunt Bauman (2003) polemicises against the dangers and threats of 'liquid life', 'liquid love', and 'dark times'. Left thinkers influenced by him have elaborated a critique of the 'social recession', which apparently belies our affluence and new freedoms. While ostensibly different from the jeremiads of conservatives such critiques come up with a similar cultural pessimism.

The late modern individual, we are told, is forced to live the illusion of freedom while actually being wrapped in the gilded cords of late capitalism and seduced by the wiles of a globalising consumer capitalism, making the most precious human bonds impossible (Hennessy 2000; Binnie 2004; Elliott and Lemert 2006). In a further refinement, critics of neo-liberalism argue that ideas of individual autonomy and responsibility of self are not so much illusory or deceptive as the very forms of regulation, which can be most effectively articulated with the current form of capitalist organisation. Neo-liberalism is the ideological face of globalising forces, undermining welfare policies that protect the individual against the depredations of international capital (see Weeks 2007: Chapter 6). As applied to sexuality and intimacy, the critiques of neo-liberalism often deploy a particular reading of the work of Michel Foucault (e.g. Rose 1999; cf. Weeks 2005), which stresses the discursive construction of subjectivities within specific regimes of power. From this perspective, neo-liberalism can be seen as a new form of governance through which the individual is, in Rose's phrase, 'forced to be free' (Rose 1999), to manage him or her self. These tendencies, it is argued, have been implicit in sexual-social policy since the Wolfenden report of 1957, but have become dominant in this period of late modernity and risk society. Under neo-liberal imperatives, individuals become 'entrepreneurs of themselves, shaping their own lives through the choices they make among the forms of life available to them' (Rose 1999: 230). This elaborate and sophisticated form of subjectivity or subjectification does not, however, lead to the abandonment of governance; it substitutes self-governance as the principle form of social regulation.

Recent liberalising sex reforms can be read in this light. Critics of same sex marriage have seen it as a move toward creating the respectable gay as opposed to the transgressive, disruptive, and challenging queer (Weeks 2007, Chapter 7). Respectability would involve a voluntary regulation of the sexual self in the interests of full acceptance and citizenship (Richardson 2004: 393). Some have seen this process working its way through the management of HIV in the 'post-crisis' world (in the West at least). A surveillance medicine, based on risk rationality, replaces hospital medicine with the aim of creating self-reflexive, self-managing subjects. People with HIV learn to calculate and manage risk, using their knowledge of their HIV status, their T cell count, blood viral load count, and the likelihood of infection to negotiate sexual partnerships (Adkins 2002: 108ff; Davis 2005: 251).

From this position the self-reflexive person is the ideal subject of neo-liberal discourse, and 'reflexivity is constitutive of new forms of classification, hierarchies, divisions, struggle and forms of contestation' (Adkins 2002: 123). An emphasis on individual freedom and rights and the importance of self-surveillance and self-regulation for the individual who has internalised the norms and goals of liberal forms of governance are central to the new society (Richardson 2004: 393). In the contemporary world they are all the more potent for seeming to be dispersed, underplayed, and voluntarily chosen.

These are seductive arguments, especially for someone like me who has been schooled in Foucauldianism. But for someone, also like me, who has lived the changes of the past few generations as well as researched and written about them, it sometimes appears that theory has become completely detached from a lived reality. Are we not genuinely freer? Do we not have more control over our lives? Are the laws not fairer? Trapped within our ideological enclosures we are in danger of failing to understand both the past and this historic present in which we live. We seem destined to be locked into alternative determinisms. A naïve progressivism, a sort of Whig interpretation of sexual history which can only see progress towards some Eden in the future, has long lost any resonance. But it is in danger of being replaced by a declinist vision, which sees a paradise lost in the past, or by a strange *mélange* of arguments – from neo-marxists, feminists, queer theorists – which seem to believe that nothing has really changed at all. None of these positions seem to me to be very convincing. The progressive myth all too readily forgets the contingencies of history, the tangled roads that have brought us to the present. The declinist myth celebrates a history that never was, a world that was not so much lost as nostalgically re-imagined to act as a counterpoint to the present. The continuists want to stress the recalcitrance of hidden structures, but in doing so forget the power of agency and the significance of subtle cumulative changes in individual lives (Weeks 2007: 4–7).

Above all, in various ways these positions obscure what seems to me the most important story: that the world we have won has made possible ways of life that represent an improvement not a decline in the conditions of sexual and intimate life. I believe the long revolution to have been overwhelmingly beneficial to the vast majority of people in the West, and increasingly to people living in the global south whose lives are also being transformed dramatically – I say that while acknowledging the major problems, inequalities, prejudices, and discriminations that remain. But the momentum, I argue, is positive, largely because of one essential feature of this new world: the power of grass-roots agency. Collective struggles – of feminism and lesbian and gay movements especially – have contributed to and complemented, but also often obscured, the reality of myriads of individual struggles by women and men over many years to gain control over the conditions of their lives. Such struggles include controlling fertility, entering in freely chosen relations, escaping oppressive relations, challenging sexual ignorance, battling against sexual violence, affirming sexual identities, having sexual pleasure, and avoiding sexual pain. These have been, in Giddens' (1992) phrase, 'everyday experiments' in which people have muddled through, making things up as they go along, living and letting live, to create the conditions for post-traditional ways of life. Increasingly, I would argue, the contemporary world is a world we are making for ourselves, part of the long process of the democratisation of everyday life. Of course that process is uneven, affecting different people at different times and places, and I will outline the balance of losses and gains later. But that does not alter the fundamental fact that the social, cultural, and moral revolution of our times is a revolution from below, and its future lies in our own hands. Unless we grasp this we cannot understand not only the problems and anxieties, but the challenges and opportunities in this world we are remaking.

The ways we lived then

To understand the changes which have transformed the world of sexuality and intimacy we need a real sense of the historicity of these changes. We live history and we are in the midst of a living history. Without a sense of history and an understanding of the ways we lived in the past, we lack benchmarks by which to measure change and the means to grasp the magnitude of the dramatic shifts that have taken place over the past 60 years.

To understand the past we have to re-imagine it without mythologising it. Like Peter Hennessy (2006) placing himself as a young observer and reflective adult in the world of the 1950s, I have found it useful to see myself as a subject of these changes. In the first place, I want to recreate the culture I was born into, of the Rhondda Valleys in South Wales in the 1940s. Historians and demographers have seen Britain's dominant patterns of family, sexuality, and fertility as belonging to a long-entrenched North West Europe model that is organised around deferred marriage, separate conjugal households, low and stable rates of illegitimacy, sexual restraint and constraint, and, from the first decades of the twentieth century, rapidly falling fertility (Szreter 2002). But that history masks separate histories, different traditions, a variety of sexual and family cultures. The South Wales Valleys mining culture I was born into had long differed from the typical pattern prevalent in much of Britain. The Welsh, says Szreter (1999: 163), 'appear to have behaved more like the French, the antithesis of the English model'. Couples married younger and had more children, and as fertility began to decline from the 1920s, they showed even more enthusiasm for marriage. There was a marked and highly gendered division of labour with few opportunities for women's employment outside the home. Women's identities were overwhelmingly bound by their domestic roles, while male culture was distinctly patriarchal and separate. Moral codes were governed by a strong religious tradition (in the Welsh case this was nonconformist) which bore down especially strongly on women's sexuality. However, there was also a popular bawdiness and a surprisingly pragmatic attitude towards, for example, abortion (Weeks 2007: 23–33). Even many decades later, while showing quite dramatic changes in sexual and family patterns, South Wales remained different from England and Wales as a whole. In the 1990s people still married younger, were more likely to marry as teenagers, and gender segregation continued to be more extreme than elsewhere: a legacy of a long history (Rees 1994; Betts 1994).

The culture was shaped around an intense sense of community and pride in place and identity. The hardships and solidarities of coal-mining above all gave the place its special ethos, especially its sense of itself as a community, and self-image as a good place to live despite its hardships. 'Community', as a dense network of kin, neighbours, friends, and community organisations, had a long resonance in the Rhondda as an essential part of its political and moral imaginary (Charles and Aull Davies 2005: 672–90; see also Chapter 9 this volume). This was a community of intense family life overlapping with a strong sense of neighbourhood so that kin and locality often merged. Whatever the blood, marital, or friendship links were, the domestic unit was based on a rigid division of labour which seemed a law of nature. Being able to maintain your family properly was a matter of male pride. Failure to do so was deeply shaming; it was effectively emasculating. In 1935 the Rhondda MP, W. H. Mainwaring, put the position with stark clarity in the context of protests against unemployment and the hated means test: 'They wanted security for their homes, sustenance for their wives. If they were not prepared to strike a blow for these things then they were not fit to be called men' (quoted in O'Leary 2004: 265). But home was different. Presiding over it was the mythical figure of the Welsh mam: stern defender of their daughters' chastity and their sons' sensitivities and needs. The mam was a 'tidy' wife who held the family together through thick and thin. As Pilcher showed in her interviews with three generations of South Wales women in the early 1990s, older women in their seventies still saw their identities as intimately bound by traditionalist views, and their daughters and grand-daughters found it difficult to escape them (Pilcher 1994).

The couples married in the 1940s, the parents of the baby boomers, were less restricted by nonconformist values than their predecessors. They were more open to the alternative visions opened up by cinema, radio, and, from the early 1950s, television. Gradually, they also had greater freedom of travel in the dawning age of affluence. The valleys were open-ing up, and older values were weakening. By the 1950s chapels were closing in every village in the Rhondda. Yet the core values and mores remained socially conservative. And it was difficult, especially, to think outside the heterosexual mould.

Homosexuality existed, but never as a distinctive way of life. It was subtly crafted into the heterosexual dynamic. Leo Abse was the Labour MP for a South Wales seat and one of the authors of the Sexual Offences Act, which partially decriminalised male homosexuality in 1967. Abse saw in the gender order one of the likely 'causes' of homosexuality in the area, which he thought endemic. The dominance of 'mam' in the family, he once told me, deploying his usual crude Freudianism, produced a large number of homosexuals, 'mammy's boys', in the valleys. He wrote else-where that 'excessive attachment to the mother can be evoked and encouraged by too much tenderness on the part of the mother herself and can be significantly reinforced by the small part played by the father during the boy's childhood' (Abse 1973: 155).

Abse's explanation is theoretically dubious. (My personal experience cer-tainly does not bear out the theory that there were hordes of homosexual men in the Rhondda when I was growing up. In fact I did not knowingly meet one till I left home and achieved a little more sexual sophistication at university in London.) However, there is no doubt that homosexuals' public presence was limited, and their space for self-identification was narrow. The obvious candi-dates for suspect homosexuality conformed to a pattern of effeminate men and butch women that is common in highly gender-segregated societies. Homosexuality was lived in the secret byways, or in exile.

The legacy remains. When in 2006 the first statistics for same-sex civil partnerships appeared there was little surprise that the Rhondda was in the bottom ten of registration districts for the number of partnerships contracted (Weeks 2007: 188). But on reflection what was perhaps more surprising was that eleven same-sex couples had 'got married' in the first six weeks. It was not so much the numbers but the fact that it had happened at all which signalled the real change. Even in the most recalcitrant areas of Britain, the iceberg was melting.

Beckoning towards freedom

South Wales had its distinct family and sexual culture, yet its characteristic moral code was echoed across Britain. It was a code based on restraint and denial. When I tell my students that up to the 1960s single mothers were still bundled into Mothers and Babies homes to escape the shame of illegitimacy, that all forms of male homosexuality were illegal, that you could end up in prison for 'the other love', and that if you were rash enough to try to commit suicide and survived you could be tried and imprisoned for a criminal offence, they laugh with disbelief. Until the 1960s Britain had some of the most draconian legal penalties against sexual nonconformity in the world. Today it has one of the most liberal legal regimes and a high degree of tolerance of sexual diversity.

This is because between the 1960s and the 1990s Britain, like most other parts of the Western world, underwent a historic transition in sexual beliefs and intimate behaviour. There was no single cause, no regular pattern across regions and countries, no common agenda for its main actors (chiefly members of the baby-boom generation). The process was messy, contradictory, and haphazard. But in the end it drew in and involved millions of people, re-imagining and remaking their lives in a myriad different ways. But the beginnings were ambiguous and uncertain. In her memoir of the 1960s, Sheila Rowbotham (2001), one of the founding mothers of second wave feminism, has written powerfully and evocatively of the sense of being poised between two worlds as the decade opens. For the young women giving birth to a child out of wedlock and surrendering it straight away to adoption, there was still a heartbreaking contradiction between the hope of greater freedom and the cultural and economic pulls of respectability and sheer necessity. The young woman tentatively embracing a sexual career soon found that social taboos and practical means lagged well behind desire. For a long time the fear of the consequences of incautious sexual practices continued to haunt individual activity (Rowbotham 2001: 48).

For the closeted homosexual, too, the promises opened up by the more sex-positive mood of the early 1960s largely remained dreams deferred. Law reform beckoned distantly, but the fear of exposure, the developing threat of aversion therapy, or what the imminent gay liberation movement would label as 'internalised self oppression' continued to haunt everyday life. In 1964 and 1965 the liberal journalist Brian Magee presented two television programmes on the 'One in Twenty' alleged to be homosexual (Magee 1966), during which the homosexual interviewees' faces remained shrouded in shadows. 'Living in the shadows' was to remain the dominant metaphor for the homosexual, male or female, until the 1970s.

For many, then, the 1960s remained a decade of unfulfilled hopes. Yet within barely a generation, the old shadows had been dispersed and replaced by quite new shapes and configurations. In the early 1990s, following more than a decade of highly conservative government, the question of single parenthood became the focus of political controversy and of cultural anxiety again, but this time one-parent families numbered nearly two million and could not easily be gainsaid; the stigma of illegitimacy was disappearing from the statute book as well as everyday life. Similarly, by the 1990s, in the wake of the AIDS epidemic, no one could have been in any doubt about who gay men were and what they did after endless documentaries and media coverage of risky behaviour and the increasing 'outness' of prominent public figures. In little more than 30 years, before the baby boomers had reached middle age, the sexual world had been irretrievably transformed and attitudes to marriage or non-marriage, childbearing or non-parenting, female sexuality, family, and sexual unorthodoxy had all changed fundamentally. Abortion and homosexuality had been at least partially decriminalised and followed by dramatic shifts in behaviour and attitudes. Divorce law had been modestly reformed but the results were dramatically immodest. The obscenity laws had been mildly reformulated but within a decade people were speaking alarmingly of floods of pornography. Theatre censorship by the archaic office of the Lord Chamberlain was abolished, contraception on the NHS was made universal, lone parent benefits were introduced, tax benefits for married couples had been drastically reduced, non-heterosexual families of choice were becoming commonplace, and same sex parenting, adoption, and marriage were appearing on the agenda.

Between the 1960s and the 1990s there were profound shifts in the social relations of sexuality and intimacy. Amongst the most important are: a shift of power between the generations; a shift in power between men and women; the separation of sex and reproduction; the separation of sex and marriage; the separation of marriage and parenting; and a redefinition of the relationship between 'normality' and 'abnormality'. Together they led, over this period of the Great Transition from the 1960s to the 1990s, to the effective demise of the traditional model of sexual restraint, and opened the way to a new moral economy. This new moral economy was less hierarchical and more democratic, hedonistic, individualistic, and selfish, perhaps, but also vastly more tolerant, experimental, and open to diversity and choice in a way that had been inconceivable just a generation earlier.

A new world arising

In a very useful exercise, Plummer (2003: 10) has attempted to balance the different ways of seeing these changes: widening disparities between rich and poor can be set against higher standards of living for most, if not all; social fragmentation can be read as a 'pluralisation' of life chances; impersonality and loss of community may be set against a new sense of belonging in new sexual worlds; narcissism and selfishness must be measured against a proliferation of new individual freedoms; McDonaldisation and standardisation have to be seen against a proliferation of choices in the democracy of the market place; dumbing down is matched by a sophisticated self-awareness, an ironic reflexivity; moral decline can be countered by a definite moral effervescence and global citizenship; entrenched hierarchies of exclusion are met with the language of inclusion and belonging, and a deepening democratisation of everyday life; and uncertainty and risk are set against the possibilities of a new global order and global human rights.

Both sides of the dichotomies may be true. The reality is that this is a world that has lost the unifying myths, the grand story which linked gender, sexuality, and family into a more or less coherent unity sanctified by Church, State, and community values. That world was never quite what it claimed to be, and in many ways was, I have suggested, as fractured and divided as our contemporary world. Yet its unifying myths did provide a sort of glue that held the structures together. Today that glue has dissolved. The power of traditional authorities, religion, family, conventional morality, and even ideology, have been battered by decades of challenge and change. They have been eroded by the dissolving powers of global flows, economic modernisation, and cultural transformations, as well as by the will for change represented by the everyday choices of countless millions. Today, we live in a plural world, a world of irreducible diversity and multiple sources of authority.

How, then, do we draw up a balance sheet? In what follows I weigh the pluses and minuses against one another to show the ambivalence as well as the reality of positive change.

The 'gender revolution'

The position of women remains the most sensitive marker of deep-structured change. On all such markers – of education, employment opportunities, family roles, and reproductive and sexual choice – there have been major shifts. The category of gender itself has been fundamentally challenged by the emergence of movements of transgendered people (Ekins and King 2006). The gender order (Connell 1987, 1995, 2002) has been shaken, and even destabilised. But the impact of the changes has been uneven, especially on a global scale. The Equal Opportunities Commission starkly stated in July 2007 that in the UK sex discrimination remained rife and full equality could take generations (Carvel 2007: 7). Even the most self-confident women still hear the 'male in the head' (Holland *et al*. 1998) calling them back to sexual subordination. Even the most enlightened men find it difficult to cast off their privileges. We remain locked in relationships of superiority and subordination at various levels. Violence and abuse still police the boundaries.

There have been many factors underlying the transformations of relations between men and women, but a key one has been the dramatic changes in the social relations of reproduction. There was birth control before the Pill, and dramatic falls in the birth rate before the 1970s, but the Pill, as a female-controlled and relatively reliable contraceptive, helped both realise and symbolise a massive, world-historic shift: the separation of sex and reproduction (McLaren 1999, Chapter 4; Cook 2005). As time has moved on it has become clear that the issue of reproductive rights has wider resonances: the right to have children as well as not; the right to terminate pregnancies in defined situations as well as to go ahead with them; and the right to control and enhance fertility. There are also complex issues about non-traditional means of conception and the rights of non-heterosexual parents. Above all, there are fundamental questions of access to resources, power, and opportunity on a global scale (Petchesky 2003).

What has genuinely shifted, however, are the fundamental terms of the debate. The story is not so much that men and women are now equal or treated equally. The real achievement is that inequality has lost all its moral justification. Inequality now has to be justified in ways it never had to be before. The fact that traditional differences now have to be rewritten in terms of equality is a measure of how far things have come (if also, at times, an index of how far there is still to go).

The coming out of homosexuality

As the heterosexual nexus linking gender order, family, and sexual reproduction has changed, so homosexuality has come out of the shadows. The sharp binary schism between heterosexuality and homosexuality that has structured, defined, and distorted the Western sexual regime for the past couple of centuries, and perhaps reached a peak in the final determined reassertion of the domestic ideology of the 1950s, has been fundamentally undermined as millions of gays and lesbians, bisexuals and transgendered people have not so much subverted the established order as lived as if their sexual difference did not matter (Adam *et al*. 1999a and b; Altman 2001). Perhaps the most significant evidence of this is the growing toleration of homosexuality in most Western countries. No longer a sin or a sickness, but barely a transgression, with same sex marriage apparently the key issue in many jurisdictions, LGBT lives are in danger of becoming ordinary (Weeks

2007: 198). But never underestimate the importance of being ordinary, especially when considering cultures in which homosexuality remains trapped in regimes of abnormality and homophobia remains rife.

It is simultaneously possible to acknowledge the transformed possibilities of living a non-heterosexual life in most parts of the urban, highly-developed world while recognising the profound continuing weight of heteronormative values and structures. Homosexuality may have come out into the open and have made institutionalised heterosexuality porous, but even in the advanced cultures of the West it is still subjected to the minoritising forces that excluded it in the first place. In other parts of the world social obloquy, long imprisonment and even death (by stoning or beheading) remain the fate of many homosexual people (Bamforth 2005). For far too many that face of Otherness remains shrouded in mystery and fear; the result is a terror that makes homosexuality an impossible way of life.

A 'transformation of intimacy'

The gender revolution and the challenge to heteronormativity are under-pinned and accelerated by a profound change in the ways in which men and women, men and men, and women and women relate to each other. The transformation of intimacy, its main proponent argues (Giddens 1992), is towards egalitarian, open, and disclosive relationships which are marked by the 'pure relationship'. Same sex relationships have been seen as especially important to this transformation, leading the way to more egalitarian forms of relationships and creative life experiments, as much by force of circum-stances as design (Weeks et al. 2001). There are many critics of this position (Jamieson 1998, 1999), and the most we can perhaps say is that the evi-dence remains uncertain and uneven. But behind the controversies there does seem to be a longer-term trend towards informalisation and democra-tisation of intimate life that is a revolution in everyday life. As yet the trend has unrealised and unsettling implications for the relationship between pri-vate passions and public life (Wouters 2004, Weeks 2007: 63–72).

A critical aspect of this process is the changing nature of family life. The apparent decline of the traditional family is frequently seen as the marker, cause, and consequence of changes in sexual relationships, childbearing, the decline of marriage, and so on. Its decay is blamed for the weakening of social capital – those norms, values, and networks that are held to sustain social trust and stability (Fukuyama 1999; Edwards 2004). Yet there is another story of: diversification of family forms caused by a weakening of patriarchal authority over women and children; the emergence of a more complex and diverse culture as a result of mass immigration; and the sheer pluralisation of household patterns and domestic arrangements – which themselves include stories of cohabitation and the decline of (heterosexual) marriage, single parenthood, the growth of people living on their own (see

Chapter 11 this volume), the emergence of serial monogamy as the dominant form of sexual partnering, and the rise of non-heterosexual (and of heterosexual) 'families of choice' that are underpinned by the 'friendship ethic' (Lewis 2001; Weeks *et al.* 2001). All of these justify the claim that we should talk about families rather than the family, recognise and appreciate the varied ways of doing family-like things, and celebrate the emergence of new and diverse forms of reciprocity, relationships, and social capital, rather than lament the decline of the family.

The irresistible rise of sexual diversity

Gayle Rubin (1984) famously spoke of the advance of the perverse sexualities out of the pages of Krafft-Ebing onto the stage of history. Today the very category of the perverse has all but disappeared. People not only proudly proclaim their gayness, bisexuality, sado-masochisms, trans-identities, fetishisms, and fantasies in all their infinite variety, but they can satisfy them through the infinite possibilities of the Internet. We dwell in a world of polymorphous non-perversities (Giddens 1992). But this is only a part of the radical diversity that characterises contemporary life. There are different ways of life, shaped by 'race' and ethnicity, class and geography, age, (dis)ability, and so on. There are also, as Gilroy (2004) has argued, new forms of 'conviviality' which defy such simple categorisations and can be said to represent the fraying of difference, if not yet the disappearance of divisions.

A proliferation of sexual stories

As this suggests we can now tell our sexual stories in a huge variety of different ways. Michel Foucault (1979) wrote of the discursive explosion since the eighteenth century which produced sexual modernity. But that was defined by rules on who could speak, in what circumstances and on whose authority. Now we can hear everyone who wants to speak, and can access means of speaking, speak their truths. Venues include everything from talk shows to home movies, from parliaments to the media, and from the streets to personal blogs, as well as interactive, user-generated sites on the Internet. Through stories – of desire and love, of hope and mundane reality, of excitement and disappointment – told to willing listeners in communities of meaning, people imagine and re-imagine who and what they are and what they want to become (Plummer 1995, 2003). Now there are many would-be authorities competing cacophonously, especially in the anarchic democracy of cyber-space. By no means are all of these voices progressive by any definition of the word; some voices are evangelical Christian or radical Islamicist, and they are as loud as any liberal or libertarian voices. There are threats as well as opportunities in the hyper market of speech. But we can no longer doubt the power of narratives, and the ways in which we can make and remake ourselves through them in the new age of globalisation (Altman 2001; Plummer 2003).

Risk and the threat of sexual disease

If we can see the globalisation of sexuality as a reordering of risk, then at the heart of the risks facing the world today is the inexorable presence and spread of the HIV/Aids pandemic (Altman 2001). Twenty years ago it was possible to largely write about it as an appalling threat to the gay populations of North America, Europe, and Australasia. Today the wealthy countries have found ways of controlling the spread of the epidemic and of managing the progression of the virus. But globally the statistics, and behind them the realities of everyday life, are terrifying. Here sexuality has become entwined in the nexus of poverty, ignorance, fear, and prejudice on a massive scale. Unlike anything else, this pandemic reveals the impossibility of separating the sexual and the intimate from the other social forces and inevitable flows of an increasingly globalised world; sexual experiences and tragedies go from nation to nation, continent to continent. Aids has become the symbol, if not the only example, of the risks of rapid sexual change in a world uncertain of its values and responses.

Culture wars

Uncertainty breeds conflict, the danger of culture wars, and the rise of both secular and religious fundamentalisms. Fundamentalisms especially can be seen as a response to uncertainty, confronting the ambiguities and ambivalences of the world with an absolute certainty about Truth, History, and Tradition (Ruthven 2004). As many have pointed out, the various forms of fundamentalism, whether Islamic, Christian, Hindu, or Jewish, are not really cultural throwbacks. They are very much products of late modernity, utilising its technologies and global linkages brilliantly (Bhatt 1997). But they are against what they see as the deformations of late modern cultures, and at the heart of these are sexuality, gender, and the body. The fundamentalisms of our time seek to restore demarcations between men and women, reaffirm heterosexual relationships, and extirpate perversity. In the most extreme manifestations they enforce their will through the bullet, the knife, and the hangman's noose. Although the tone and the tenor might be different, the religious and socially conservative movements of the USA, in their affirmation of traditional values and opposition to abortion, homosexuality, same sex marriage, sex education, evolutionism, and the like, share some common assumptions with fundamentalisms: a belief that there is an essential truth to sexuality for which they know the key. Culture wars are the inevitable result.

The making of sexual/intimate citizenship

It is in this context that new discourses about sexual or intimate citizenship have emerged (Plummer 1995, 2003). Citizenship is about belonging, recognition, and reciprocal entitlements and responsibilities. Historically, citizenship has been restricted – racially, xenophobically, and by gender and sexuality (Brandzel 2005). We forget how recent has been the achievement of full citizenship rights for women, how restrictive were the assumptions behind the Welfare State's structure of entitlements, and how minorities and 'deviants' were excluded from the rights and obligations of full citizenship. Sexual or intimate citizenship is about the recognition of these exclusions and the moves to inclusion (Weeks 1998; Bell and Binnie 2000; Richardson 2000a and b; Plummer 2003). The steps in the process have been erratic, and in many jurisdictions, including the most wealthy and most powerful, are not yet fully realised. Yet without the idea of full citizenship we cannot measure how far we have come; and without the ideal of equal citizenship we have no measure of how far we still have to go.

This becomes especially challenging in the context of globalisation and 'global sex' (Altman 2001). Sexuality has a 'central significance within global regimes of power' (Hemmings *et al.* 2006: 1), and this is manifest in persistent inequities between cultures and continuing sexual injustices, especially against women, children, and lesbian, gay, or transgendered identified peoples. At the same time, we see the emergence of global standards of what constitutes justice. We can learn to accept difference and human variety, including various ways of being sexual, and this has become a new imperative as we get to know more and more about other cultures. We can understand the power differentials that underpin difference. But increasingly, in a world not just of different but conflicting values, many people are also seeking common standards by which to measure behaviours. We have become aware of sufferings across the world where 'before they might have gone unnoticed' (Baird 2004: 8). We can no longer easily fail to notice when the survivors of injustices can tell us of their sufferings across the globalised media, from the Internet to television, and when waves of people begin to appear at our own doorsteps, seeking refuge from persecution. Globalisation has made us aware of sexual wrongs across the world, and has awakened us to the significance of sexual rights. As Nussbaum (1999: 8) has persuasively argued, a universal account of human justice need not be insensitive to the variety of traditions that shape human lives, nor is it a mere projection of particular Western values onto parts of the world with different concerns. The evolution of human sexual rights has been a process that engages the Other and involves a dialogue across differences. The concept of sexual rights that is emerging provides space and opportunity for difference to flourish within a developing discourse of our common humanity.

Conclusion

This is a long way from small mining valleys in South Wales where I began my personal story and this particular analysis. And yet that local history was already caught up in a much larger history of 'coal as king', of empire, of different sexual cultures, and of family and gendered identities. All of these histories complexly interacted to create a way of life that shaped generations; they shaped me, even as I have spent a lifetime escaping from it and attempting to do it differently. In the melancholia of a post-colonial world (Gilroy 2004) it is all too easy to forget how much has been gained.

It has become a cliché that sexuality has a history, indeed many histories. But it is easy to forget, as we live our own sexual history, that alongside us people are living theirs, and their experience might be quite different from ours. And as I write I cannot help reflecting that I am already constructing a 'we' that is distinguishing my group from yours and theirs. I am already heavily engaged in Othering, which is a key process in the construction of sexualities. What a historical approach to sexuality can do is make us aware of our commonalities and differences. It should alert us to the ways in which the erotic is shaped in complex relations of power. It should also make us aware of our contingency.

No one in 1945 could have foreseen the world we now inhabit and have helped to remake. We live in a different world. But if we forget our history we are in danger of having to re-live it. Perhaps one of the greatest achievements of the long revolution is that it has made us reflexive, sensitive to our own historicity and to the profoundly challenging notion that if we have made our own history we can also remake it. That may, in the end, be the most important reason for attempting a history of the world we have won.

References

Abse, L (1973) *Private Member*, London: Macdonald.

Adam, B. D., Duyvendak, J. W. and Krowell, A. (eds) (1999a) *The Global Emergence of Gay and Lesbian Politics: National Imprints of a Wordwide Movement*, Philadelphia, PA: Temple University Press.

Adam, B. D., Duyvendak, J. W. and Krowell, A. (eds) (1999b) 'Gay and Lesbian Movements Beyond Borders? National Imprints of a Wordwide Movement', in Adam, B. D., Duyvendak, J. W. and Krowell, A. (eds) (1999) *The Global Emergence of Gay and Lesbian Politics: National Imprints of a Wordwide Movement*, Philadelphia, PA: Temple University Press.

Adkins, L. (2002) *Revisions: Gender and Sexuality in Late Modernity*, Buckingham: Open University Press.

Altman, D. (2001) *Global Sex*, Chicago: University of Chicago Press.

Baird, V. (2004) *Sex, Love and Homophobia: Lesbian, Gay, Bisexual and Transgender Lives*, London: Amnesty International.

Bamforth, N. (2005) *Sex Rights*, Oxford Amnesty Lectures, Oxford and New York: Oxford University Press.

Bauman, Z. (2003) *Liquid Love: On the Frailty of Human Bonds*, Cambridge: Polity Press.

Bell, D. and Binnie, J. (2000) *The Sexual Citizen: Queer Politics and Beyond*, Cambridge: Polity Press.

Betts, S. (1994) 'The Changing Family in Wales', in Aaron, J., Rees, T., Betts, S. and Vincentelli, M. (eds) *Our Sisters' Land: The Changing Identities of Women in Wales*, Cardiff: University of Wales Press.

Bhatt, C. (1997) *Liberation and Purity: Race, New Religious Movements and the Ethics of Postmodernity*, London: University College London Press.

Binnie, J. (2004) *The Globalization of Sexuality*, London and Thousand Oaks, New Delhi: Sage Publications.

Brandzel, A. L. (2005) 'Queering Citizenship? Same-sex Marriage and the State', *GLQ: A Journal of Lesbian and Gay Studies* 11(2): 171–204.

Carvel, J. (2007) 'Sex discrimination rife and equality will take generations, says axed commission', *The Guardian*, 24 July, 7.

Charles, N. and Aull Davies, C. (2005) 'Studying the Particular, Illuminating the General: Community Studies and Community in Wales', *Sociological Review* 53(4), November: 672–90.

Connell, R. W. (1987) *Gender and Power*, Cambridge: Polity Press.

Connell, R. W. (1995) *Masculinities*, Cambridge: Polity Press.

Connell, R. W. (2002) *Gender*, Cambridge: Polity Press.

Cook, H. (2005) *The Long Sexual Revolution: English Women, Sex, and Contraception 1800–1975*, Oxford: Oxford University Press.

Davies, C. (2006) *The Strange Death of Moral Britain*, New York: Transaction Publishers.

Davis, M. D. M. (2005) *Treating and Preventing HIV in the Post-crisis situation: Perspectives from the Personal Experience Accounts of Gay Men with HIV*, unpublished PhD thesis, Institute of Education, University of London.

Duncan Smith, I. (2007) *Breakdown Britain*, Social Justice Policy Group, Centre for Social Justice.

Edwards, R. (2004) 'Present and Absent in Troubling Ways: Families and Social Capital Debates', *The Sociological Review* 52(1), February: 1–21.

Ekins, R. and King, D. (2006) *The Transgender Phenomenon*, London and Thousand Oaks, New Delhi: Sage.

Elliott, A. and Lemert, C. (2006) *The New Individualism: The Emotional Costs of Globalization*, London and New York: Routledge.

Foucault, M. (1979) *The History of Sexuality: Volume 1: An Introduction*, Harmondsworth: Penguin.

Fukuyama, F. (1999) *The Great Disruption: Human Nature and the Reconstitution of Social Order*, London: Profile Books.

Giddens, A. (1992) *The Transformation of Intimacy: Sexuality, Love and Eroticism in Modern Societies*, Cambridge: Polity Press.

Gilroy, P. (2004) *After Empire: Melancholia or Convivial Culture*, London: Routledge.

Hemmings, C., Gedalof, I. and Bland, L. (2006) 'Sexual Moralities', *Feminist Review* 83, 1–3.

Hennessy, P. (2006) *Having it so Good: Britain in the Fifties*, London: Allen Lane.

Hennessy, R. (2000) *Profit and Pleasure: Sexual Identities in Late Capitalism*, New York and London: Routledge.

Holland, J., Ramazanoglu, C., Sharpe, S. and Thomson, R. (1998) *The Male in the Head*, London: The Tufnell Press.

Jamieson, L. (1998) *Intimacy: Personal Relationships in Modern Societies*, Polity Press, Cambridge.

Jamieson, L. (1999) 'Intimacy Transformed: A Critical Look at the "Pure Relationship"', *Sociology* 33(3): 447–94.

Laslett, P. (1965) *The World We Have Lost*, London: Methuen.

Lewis, J. 2001 *The End of Marriage? Individualism and Intimate Relations*, Cheltenham and Northampton, MA: Edward Elgar.

Magee, B. (1966) *One in Twenty*, London: Secker and Warburg.

McLaren, A. (1999) *Twentieth-Century Sexuality: A History*, Oxford: Blackwell.

Nussbaum, M. (1999) *Sex and Social Justice*, New York and Oxford: Oxford University Press.

O'Leary, P. (2004) 'Masculine Histories: Gender and the Social History of Modern Wales', *Welsh History Review* 22(2): 252–77.

Petchesky, R. (2003) 'Negotiating Reproductive Rights', in Weeks, J., Holland, J. and Waites, M. (eds) *Sexualities and Society: A Reader*, Cambridge: Polity Press.

Phillips, M. (1999) *The Sex-change Society: Feminised Britain and Neutered Male*, London: The Social Market Foundation.

Pilcher, J. (1994) 'Who Should Do the Dishes? Three Generations of Welsh Women Talking about Men and Housework', in Aaron, J., Rees, T., Betts, S. and Vincentelli, M. (eds.) *Our Sisters' Land: The Changing Identities of Women in Wales*, Cardiff: University of Wales Press.

Plummer, K. (1995) *Telling Sexual Stories: Power, Change and Social Worlds*, London: Routledge.

Plummer, K. (2003) *Intimate Citizenship: Private Decisions and Public Dialogues*, Seattle: University of Washington Press.

Rees, T. (1994) 'Women and Paid Work in Wales', in Aaron, J., Rees, T., Betts, S. and Vincentelli, M. (eds) *Our Sisters' Land: The Changing Identities of Women in Wales*, Cardiff: University of Wales Press.

Richardson, D. (2000a) *Rethinking Sexuality*, London and Thousand Oaks, New Delhi: Sage.

Richardson, D. (2000b) 'Claiming Citizenship? Sexuality, Citizenship and Lesbian/Feminist Theory', *Sexualities* 3(2), May: 255–72.

Richardson, D. (2004) 'Locating Sexualities: From Here to Normality', *Sexualities* 7(4): 391–411.

Rose, N. (1999) *Governing the Soul: The Shaping of the Private Self*, 2nd edition, London and New York: Free Associations Books.

Rowbotham, S. (2001) *Promise of a Dream: Remembering the Sixties*, London and New York: Verso.

Rubin, G. (1984) 'Thinking sex: notes for a radical theory of the politics of sexuality', in C.S. Vance (ed.) *Pleasure and Danger. Exploring Female Sexuality*, London and Boston: Routledge and Kegan Paul: 267–319.

Ruthven, M. (2004) *Fundamentalism: The Search for Meaning*, Oxford: Oxford University Press.

Szreter, S. (1999) 'Failing Fertilities and Changing Sexualities in Europe since c.1850: A Comparative Survey of National Demographic Patterns', in Eder, F.X., Hall, L. A. and Hekma, G. (eds) *Sexuality in Europe: Themes in Sexuality*, Manchester: Manchester University Press.

Szreter, S. (2002) *Fertility, Class and Gender in Britain, 1860–1940*, Cambridge: Cambridge University Press.

Toynbee, P. (2007) 'This broken society rhetoric leaves Cameron marooned', *The Guardian*, 10 July, 31.

Weeks, J. (1998) 'The Sexual Citizen', *Theory, Culture and Society* 15(3–4): 35–52.

Weeks, J. (2005) 'Remembering Foucault', *Journal of the History of Sexuality* 14(1/2), January/April: 186–201.

Weeks, J. (2007) *The World We Have Won: The Remaking of Erotic and Intimate Life*, London: Routledge.

Weeks, J., Heaphy, B. and Donovan, C. (2001) *Same Sex Intimacies: Families of Choice and other Life Experiments*, London: Routledge.

Wouters, C. (2004) *Sex and Manners: Female Emancipation in the West, 1890–2000*, London and Thousand Oaks, New Delhi: Sage Publications.

Chapter 5

Families in black and minority ethnic communities and social capital

Past and continuing false prophecies in social studies

Harry Goulbourne

Introduction

A crucial aspect of current academic and public debates about social exclusion concerns the integration of people who are generally regarded as new minority racial and ethnic communities into wider British society. The interest in this process is sometimes expressed in terms of the amount and quality of social capital that these minorities are said to possess and use: some groups are presumed to have high levels of social capital, while others are said to have too little, the 'wrong' kinds, or none at all. The questions which arise from this concern are not, however, new to students of trends in public policy or academic social studies over the past four or so decades. For the better part of this period policy-makers, academics, journalists, and others have been commenting upon the possible futures of community cohesion and integration. These commentators have shared a common methodology of comparing people from vastly different cultures and historical backgrounds, as well as generally focusing on a perhaps too exclusively British national context.

In this chapter, I revisit some highly influential academic observations about the ability of newcomers to integrate into British society, and set these out in terms of present debates about social capital. However, a necessary starting point is the general context in which such debates have taken, and are taking, place in the post-imperial socio-political order emerging in Britain.

The context

There are two closely related general points regarding the context of these debates to be taken into consideration. These are, first, the range of categories of people involved, and second, an indication of what may be meant by the various terms being employed, namely, the notion of community, racial and ethnic identities, social capital, and family. It is necessary to explore these general points because they are too often either taken for granted, when in fact they are highly contentious in terms of meaning, understanding and interpretation, or too abstractly stated to be of much practical use in the needy world of community life.

So far, there is a relative neglect in social studies of subsequent groups from some of these areas as well as other communities. For example, while there was an interest in Cypriot (Oakley, 1979) and Maltese (Dench, 1975) communities, after the 1970s this interest declined. Similarly, while there has been an abiding interest in the presence of key figures from the African continent, particularly West Africa but also others (e.g. Fryer, 1984; Sherwood, 1991), there has been less of a policy or academic interest in the emergence of communities of Africans within the UK. There is, therefore, a need for empirical research about the problems and concerns of some of these apparently invisible communities which could then inform policy debates about such matters as the treatment of children, social services, and how individuals and groups with recent backgrounds in Africa differ from African Caribbeans. The problem of crime and violence among black individuals in English cities is a case in point. In general, the violent killings and the use of knives and guns are associated with new waves of Jamaicans who enter the country and are involved in the illegal drugs trade. So when, in the middle of February 2007, four young men were gunned down in South London, the national debate about crime and specific communities understandably focused on Caribbeans, particularly Jamaicans. When, however, the *South London Press* (16 February, 2006: 4–5) more widely considered crime in the region, it turned out that some killers, particularly in Peckham, were from Africa. Similarly, outstanding and highly visible individuals (such as Paul Boateng) from the continent are often assumed to be of Caribbean backgrounds. With the end of the Cold War and the eastern expansion of the European Union, new patterns of immigration have been taking place across the continent, leading to renewed policy (if not yet academic) interest in the entry of East Europeans into Britain. Thus, in June 2007 the government expressed concern about 'racial tensions' in rural areas and the integration of new migrants. Rather paradoxically, therefore, while much of the present debate about new communities concerns those that became settled from the 1960s – predominantly, Caribbeans and South Asians – many of the issues being addressed today involve the newer communities as well, and this must be a challenge for both policy and social studies.

It may be suggested, however, that we do not have to look far to understand why there has been and continues to be such an apparently unproblematic concentration or focus on Caribbeans and South Asians. I have argued elsewhere (Goulbourne, 1998) that the forging of what has been generally regarded as a multicultural society in Britain, during the decades of the 1970s to the beginning of the new millennium, has been led by individuals and groups in the Asian and Caribbean communities. In other words, while there were a variety of different groups present in

Britain before the last half century, this constituted only part of the general condition for the multicultural society; after all, the multicultural society crucially involves not just its *de facto* existence, but also its recognition, or what Parekh (2002) called a 'multi-culturalist' society. In other words, while nearly all human societies are racially and ethnically diverse, and are therefore multicultural and multi-racial, only a handful of democratic societies formally recognise this, celebrate it, and try to ensure that such diversity is not the basis for domination and/or discrimination. But the multiculturalist kind of approach to understanding or promoting the perceived 'good' society involves more than the legitimate recognition of difference. The approach includes mutual respect for differences (Jenkins, 1967) and the (perhaps ultimately contradictory and illusory) attempt to find what Swann called 'a common framework of values' (Swann, 1985) that has recently been supported by such leading public figures as Gordon Brown, David Blunkett, and Trevor Phillips.

Crucially, perhaps it may be said that the struggles over issues that concerned these communities, expressed in terms of 'multiculturalism', involved negotiating their paths into whatever is perceived to constitute the 'mainstream' society, and making their concerns the concerns of all. Following C. Wright Mills' (1970) notion of people turning their 'troubles' into 'issues' – that is, generalising their daily concerns so that they become intertwined with the troubles of others – it might be suggested that Caribbeans and South Asians have sought to generalise their problems and establish alliances with various elements of the majority population. It would then appear that other new communities (for example, the Chinese), and even less the newer communities (Africans), have not (yet) been seen to make such attempts, even though the participation of individuals from these backgrounds is well known. I pose this only as a hypothesis that requires empirical investigation.

I have been loosely speaking about such factors as community, racial and ethnic identities, social capital, and family, but it is necessary briefly to indicate what I mean when I employ such a vocabulary. Concepts and definitions of social categories are important when discussing the issues of families, communities, and social capital, particularly if a comparative methodology is used, because very different kinds of social collectivities are involved. Moreover, we nearly always import particularistic or idiosyncratic notions from across the social sciences and humanities into the meanings of these concepts and categories, making it all the more necessary to offer a working understanding of how these concepts inform this discussion.

Traditionally, the institution of the family was generally thought to be the basic unit of a social order with the function of providing for the biological and social reproduction of humans. Spinning outward from the family core (whether nuclear or extended) is the kinship group – a series of networks connected by biological descent, but equally importantly by social and legal sanctions (through such acts as marriage, and such players or agencies as in-laws). While there may be general agreement with this broad understanding, the last two decades or so have witnessed a growing dissatisfaction with what many assume constitutes the institution of the family. For example, it has been suggested that the inner nucleus of the traditional family, constituted through the partnership/marriage of two adults, used to be represented as 'me + you' (a merger in which both entities lose their autonomy or separate identities). Today the representation takes the form of 'me+you+us' (three fairly distinct entities) (Furstenberg, 2005). The distinct trinity that is displacing the traditionally fused duo gives recognition to the atomisation or individualisation of intimate relationships. For some observers there is the additional factor of the gender and sexual components in these relationships (e.g. Weeks *et al.*, 2003; Weeks Chapter 4 of this volume; Plummer, 2003). Two points may be noted here: first, families are generally located within the context of wider kinship networks; second, these, in turn, are structured and operate within and constitute communities located in specific physical spaces and/or scattered across unconnected territories, such as with transnational families (Bryceson and Vuorela, 2002; Goulbourne and Chamberlain, 2001; Goulbourne, 2002).

Necessarily, therefore, communities denote kinds of social relationships. Tonnies' (1955) distinction between *gemeinschaft* and *gesellschaft* may be useful here in making the necessary connections between families, kinship groups, and communities. Where *gemeinschaft* represents communities based on living together (such as in the home, in the village, or in the country), *gesellschaft* represents communities based on legal, contract/agreement with an identifiable aim in mind (such as in a marriage, in a business company, or in an interest group). Consistent with some other nineteenth-century theorists (e.g. Weber), Tonnies' concern was to understand what made modern societies different from traditional societies, and identified the latter sense of community as being more characteristic of modern societies. Today, we tend to be more nuanced and try to avoid sharp dualities, and consequently we may be more inclined to see both senses of community asserting themselves in intimate relationships. For example, when people increasingly use the word 'partner' to describe an intimate relationship between two individuals, it may be suggested that the vocabulary from *gesellschaft* is being used to convey a *gemeinschaft* relationship, thereby undermining or questioning a dualism between 'the public' and 'the private', or domestic domains of intimate and public relationships.

The kinds of communities with which this paper is concerned exhibit racial and ethnic identities that are supposed to be distinct from the racial and ethnic identities of the majority population. While this assumption represents one level of reality, at another level this is a misrepresentation or distortion of the situation. Both racial (meaning: phenotypical differences) and ethnic (meaning: cultural values, traditions, customs, etc.) constructions of identity hide significant similarities and complicated overlapping of groups so that we must necessarily think in terms of plural, not singular, identities. Of particular significance in the British context is the fact that over the last half of the twentieth century the entry of individuals and their families, their construction, and consolidation of the new communities they have purportedly created have not resulted in communities entirely marked off by irreconcilable value systems and an absence of inter-racial mixing and mingling in terms of either of Tonnies' communities – that is, neither in living arrangements nor in formal, contractual relationships. Of course, the warnings of prominent public figures and politicians, and the support for terrorist and criminal activities in several communities are widely reported and structure much public debate; it therefore is easy to conclude that British society is divided along the lines feared by such prophets as Enoch Powell. To be sure, the identities that Asians and Caribbeans in contemporary Britain answer to or express are new, although they have antecedents. But the notion of 'Asian' disappears in the subcontinent, as does 'African Caribbean' in the Caribbean, because these are largely British constructions – whether of a colonial kind (as in East Africa) or within post-imperial island Britain. Something of the metaphor is essential to the meanings and definitions of these 'communities', and they are certainly situational. A simple or crude comparative methodology that does not take into account these kinds of complexities is likely to result in a poor social theory that distorts social reality and the sociological enterprise of attaining clarity and understanding of lived collective lives.

This provides a useful point at which to suggest how the notion of social capital might relate to families and communities, and their identities. It is generally assumed that families and communities – particularly communities demarcated by ethnic and/or racial identities – are sites rich in social capital. The vast and growing literature on social capital – its meaning, access and use, measurement, etc. – cannot be extensively entered into in a paper of this kind. However, a working definition would suggest that social capital is about largely intangible, unquantifiable resources such as informal networks and connections that are essentially social in the sense that the realisation of its use-value is observable only where the individual or the group taps into it to produce or attain desired or beneficial results. Understood in this way, it may be taken that social capital is highly instrumental, pliable, even vague and slippery to pin down, and is not always observable. Indeed, it may be said that social capital is largely recognisable by its effect; unlike material capital (machinery, minerals, money, land, buildings, etc.), social capital is largely invisible, and cannot – unlike Marx's labourer who takes his own hide to market as a commodity – be taken to the formal marketplace in exchange for other commodities. This does not mean, however, that social capital is entirely ethereal or epiphenomenal; it is real enough and some of its effects are observable.

This perspective on the notion of social capital is informed by a critical, if not sceptical, view. First, while social capital is a useful heuristic device enabling us better to understand how some groups of people are able successfully to attain their desired ends, we can identify this social capital only when it is used successfully; it is recognised *post hoc*. Groups that are judged to be successful are therefore deemed to have a good stock of social capital; unsuccessful groups are equally assumed to be lacking in social capital. Part of Marx's critique of hoarding capital (by the Spanish in the seventeenth century), was that potentially useful capital was not in circulation and therefore became rather useless; there needed to be commodities for gold as a currency to circulate in the market. I wonder whether it may not also be the case that a group (a family, a kinship network, an ethnic community, etc.) may be rich in social capital, but because the group does not mobilise or use this capital its latency renders such social capital to the status of non-importance or irrelevance. This dormancy aside, social capital identification largely appears to be a functional exercise – an understanding of social capital in this sense can therefore be rendered an exercise in tautology. What makes one group successful and another unsuccessful may very well not be the presence or absence of social capital, but extraneous factors such as the possession of wealth, education, political power, or military force. With regard to racial and ethnic minorities in Britain, the experience of differential racism may be more responsible for differential outcomes or rewards than the nature or amount of social capital that they may be said to possess. If this line of reasoning has merit, we need to be more critical about the utility of social capital, both as 'something out there in the dark' and an analytical concept.

Second, partly arising from this situation and partly arising independently, the question has to be asked whether it is not the case that one group's social capital may not be dysfunctionality for another group, depending on the socio-historical, psychological, etc. mixes of particular groups or communities and the underlying principles of the dominant or majority ethnic and racial mixes. The collectivist orientation of Asian groups, for example, has been a marked advantage for Asian immigrants during periods of entry and settlement into British society, while the individualistic orientation of Caribbeans was perceived as a disadvantage during that phase. However, now that in the first decade of a new century we are in a phase where these groups are consolidating their presence, and when cultural and social negotiation and integration with other groups are necessary, it could be argued that the individualistic orientation is more of a resource than strong in-group bonding. While internally possessing more strength through solidarity, the collectivistic orientation may be less malleable and adaptable to new and changing situations.

What, then, is social capital in one context may not be social capital in another. Thus, for example, immigrants from the Caribbean or the Punjab who came from rural backgrounds would have found their agricultural skills and networks to be of little or no use in the urban parts of England that they settled or in the new kinds of networks they needed to make a living and establish their families. On the other hand, the solidarity engineered in rural communities can be manipulated to engender networks which enable resource-deprived individuals to overcome poverty and isolation. An example of this is the Caribbean 'partnership'. This is a simple or primitive form of capital-collection more than capital-accumulation (as there is no profit nor interest) which provides financial support for members of the network, thereby overcoming the disadvantages of exclusion from financial lending institutions, such as banks and mortgage companies, in the decades from the 1950s to the 1970s.

Social capital cannot, therefore, be seen as a set of factors that can be agreed upon, unproblematically identified, and easily measured across different social groups and communities – particularly across communities which are differentiated by racial and/or ethnic identities, and have different cultural values, customs, and socio-historical and psychological compositions. This admission amounts to a critique of both the comparative method and social capital of method and theory. But while this critique does not mean an abandonment of comparative studies (and indeed quite the contrary), outlining the virtues of this Aristotelian methodology is outside the scope of this chapter. Rather, in the remainder of this chapter it is more relevant to offer some examples of how what may be regarded as social capital of ethno-racial groups can be massively misrepresented when we do not understand the basis or values of these groups' social action. And this can result in undermining sound comparative studies of racial and ethnic communities.

Past assumptions and presumptions

Assumptions and presumptions about the possession of social capital by Caribbeans and Asians are now something of a tradition in British social studies. To be sure, the vocabulary has changed from cultural strength or possession to social capital, but the substance of the assumptions and presumptions remain constant alongside a strong and unabashed tendency to endow the cultural values of one group with worth and those of the other group with deprecation. Over time, the groups change places. While this theme is replete through a body of literature, perhaps there is nowhere that it is more systematically implied than in Rex's work, particularly his *Colonial immigrants in a British city: a class analysis* (Rex and Tomlinson, 1979). Given the context described above, it was not surprising that Rex and Tomlinson's overall concerns were: first, the question of integration; second, a general desirability for peace and the avoidance of racial/ethnic conflict; and third, issues arising from the radicalism of the period characterised by questions about the Third World, world communism, and capitalism in the

West. The basic question for Rex and Tomlinson was: what are the chances for Caribbeans and Asians integrating into mainstream British society? Their answer turned out to be something along the lines of the fact that when taking racism as a constant, the immigrants' chances of successfully integrating into British society largely turn on what they arrived with in terms of their general cultural baggage, that is, language, religion, values, norms, and attitudes as well as their capacity to engage with the 'host society'. The vocabulary they and many of their contemporaries used is different from today's social capital vocabulary, but the contents and meanings are much the same: family and kinship, network and community, values and norms, attitudes, and so forth. In exploring these issues Rex and Tomlinson sensibly concentrated on specific problems faced by these communities, including housing, education, employment, and so forth – these are areas of national life with which we are still concerned today.

Speaking about the problems of children in school and the cultural baggages brought by children from the English working class and Asian and West Indian backgrounds to the school site, Rex and Tomlinson argued that:

> The West Indians are aware that they are at a disadvantage compared with the Asians, because of the strength of the Asian culture, and at a disadvantage compared with the white working class who, despite their cultural differences from their teachers, none the less do share with those teachers the fact of being English.
>
> (Rex and Tomlinson, 1979: 29)

They had stated earlier that:

> Of all the children involved in our study, the alternative of cultural bilingualism is most available to the children of Asian immigrants. Most of them have as a reference point a home culture based upon a distinct system of morals, language and religion set within a kinship structure. Parents and religious organisations will do all that they can to strengthen this culture. So far as English children are concerned, there are no such alternatives. They confront the school system with class and regional accents and the bits and pieces of a class and regional culture which survive in an urban mass society. *The West Indians have the most difficulty of all.* Their cultural history is one in which originally African culture was nearly completely destroyed by slavery, *in which they were offered an inferior position within a variant of English culture, and in which they began to develop their own culture of defiance and revolt.* It is from this complex cultural situation in West Indian homes that West Indian children come to encounter the culture of the schools.
>
> (ibid. 28, emphases added)

This theme of the inherent cultural superiority of Asians over both the white working class and West Indians is replete throughout the text – and is a theme to be found in other publications by Rex (Rex, 1970). For example, speaking of the possibility of including aspects of West Indian or black history and culture in the school curriculum, Rex and Tomlinson asserted:

> From this point of view the Asian communities must be objects of envy to the West Indian. Their religious and cultural traditions and organizations are strong, and, even while their children are using school education in an instrumental way, their supplementary cultural education confirms a worthy self-image. Moreover, the host society has learned to recognize the separate Asian religions and the West Indian is thought of as having no culture and as having no claim to have his culture taught in schools.
>
> (Rex and Tomlinson, 1979: 171)

Given the debates that have gone on and are presently going on about the contents of the history syllabus in schools, and the re-examination of the Atlantic Slave Trade as part of the commemoration of the bicentenary of its abolition in 1807, this forecast must now seem to reaffirm Hegel's aphorism that 'history teaches that history teaches nothing'.

Central to Rex and Tomlinson's argument is the inferiority or absence of West Indian culture, and the need to *invent* a culture. However, never fear, for Rastafarianism (like Black Islam and Black Power in the USA) '... will provide them [West Indians] at least with the beginnings of a culture of self-respect' (ibid. 237). They prophesied that while both Asian and West Indian young people are deprived in terms of education, employment, and housing, and this deprivation may form the basis for shared collective action, 'Together they will form an immigrant-descended social formation which, if it cannot enter the class system, will figure as an underclass to defend itself' (ibid. 237). But if there is a sense or feeling of Social Darwinism infusing this perspective – where one group has the capacity to survive in this harsh and competitive world of racism and the other group does not – these differences point to different futures for the two groups, precisely because of the quality of their cultural baggages:

> If the West Indian is plagued by self-doubt induced by white education, and seeks a culture which will give him a sense of identity, the Asians have religions and cultures and languages of which they are proud and which may prove surprisingly adaptive and suited to the demands of a modern industrial society.
>
> (ibid. 237)

The prophecy, therefore, was that:

> It is possible ... that amongst West Indians the very basis of their cul-
> ture will be one of self-assertion against white society and that this may
> be a crucial factor in turning the West Indian community into a kind of
> ethnic class-for-itself.
>
> (ibid. 171)

This kind of social analysis compares with, and must be set within, much
the same mould as that of J. Enoch Powell, who had also prophesied that
there would be 'rivers of blood' on British streets as a result of West Indian
and Asian communities springing up in British cities. Powell had also constructed a dualism of Asian cultural strength and West Indian cultural
weakness, but where Rex and Tomlinson predicted the outcome to be Asian
integration, Powell thought that 'the white man' should more fear the
Asian's cultural strength. With regard to how these communities' cultures
would enable them to engage with the 'host society', Rex and Tomlinson
turn more closely to religion, family, and kinship networks, community
organisations, and their respective attitudes and values. In a chapter entitled
'Race, community and conflict', an interesting set of diagrams illustrates the
different groups' *'deviant tendencies'* from the *norms* of British society.
Having commented at some length on these elsewhere (Goulbourne, 1990),
I want to restrict comments here to their four pointers or deviant tendencies
for community groups:

- confrontation, aggression, and black revolution
- withdrawal as practical strategy or utopian ideal
- integrationism or seeking peaceful coexistence (with the host community)
- alliance with native white radicalism.

By this point the reader of Rex and Tomlinson cannot be surprised when a
sharply drawn dichotomous general conclusion is arrived at:

> In the case of the West Indian community ... What is perhaps more
> interesting ... is that movements emphasizing black identity need to be
> placed on our diagram somewhere between practical social work, *with-
> drawal, and confrontation and aggression. Arguably, movements which
> have this theme are the most important phenomena amongst West
> Indians.*
>
> (Rex and Tomlinson, 1979: 245–6, emphasis added)

Activities by West Indian groups nearly all represent 'withdrawal' from
society and societal norms:

Thus, for example, in the diagram for West Indian religion [*sic*] one would find a place for Rastafarianism at the withdrawal corner of Figure 8.2 (b), ... but Penticostalism, on the other hand, would represent a kind of religious withdrawal, but might also be seen as having to do with a particular kind of adaptation.

(ibid. 247)

On the other hand:

In the case of the Asian groups, what one has to notice is that the core activities and all four deviant tendencies are covered from within the framework of a group based strongly on kinship, religion and ethnicity. *The withdrawal alternative means that kin ties are strengthened as a defensive measure against external threat.* The confrontation alternative is closely related as when vigilante and community defence groups are proposed. Alliance with white radicalism takes place through workers' associations which, though they may communicate in terms of socialist and Marxist theory with white groups, are also based upon kin, religious and ethnic structures. Even integration is a strategy pursued by the group as a whole and takes the form of community elites coming to terms with the representatives of the host society.

(ibid. 246, emphasis added)

There is much to comment upon in Rex and Tomlinson's work, but in great measure for any scholar with little more than a general knowledge of the groups or communities being described, the extensive references here partly speak for themselves in terms of the exercise in social distortion as a result of a reliance on uninformed perceptions and a flawed application of the comparative method, as opposed to balanced and informed social inquiry. However, it must be stressed that many of their views were shared by some of their contemporaries, and while the point needs to be more carefully researched, it is surprising that whatever voices there were against this aspect of Rexism they were rather muted.

A significant example of a work that wittingly or unwittingly reflects and reinforces Rexism is Geoff Dench's (1986) *Minorities in the open society: prisoners of ambivalence.* Dench suggests that different communities (South Asians, South Europeans, Jews, Irish, Caribbeans, and others) in Britain confront 'the open society' in one of two ways. First, in some communities (notably Jewish and Asian) leaders maintain strong internal/communalist control by manipulating material and cultural resources, thereby protecting their communities from the incapacitating onslaughts of the 'open society':

The problem is least burdensome for communities such as the Jews, or in post-war Britain most of the Asian groups. These possess the economic and cultural resources to maintain some influence over members. They may even be content to remain partially excluded, in violation of the commandment to integrate. But less coherent groups, or to put it another way those with no choice but to play by the rules that the open society decrees, and obliged to see themselves as free agents, are placed in grave peril by having their misdemeanours dragged out into public.

(Dench, 1986: 122)

This statement perceives the openness of some groups – particularly Irish and Caribbean groups – to be a weakness, and the strong communalist control by leaders in other communities to be a strength. In the wake of what is generally described in public and academic discourses as 'Muslim fundamentalism', and particularly the London suicide bombings on Thursday 7 July 2005, in the 'open' society, communalist enclaves are now perceived as likely to result in communal conflict. Indeed, paternalistic leadership which operates in the shadows is challenged not just from outside by the values (as expressed through law and mores), but also from within on a variety of bases – not least feminism, youth, and a general desire to be part of the broad stream of society.

This leads to a few general remarks about the methodological approach of the negative perspective of apportioning value and non-value to different communities in Rexian sociology. I have pointed elsewhere to the historicity of Rex's sociology (Goulbourne, 1998), particularly with respect to his more theoretical work, *Race relations in sociological theory* (1970), but this comes out particularly strongly in *Colonial immigrants*, which, after all, was meant to be a work of theory but one grounded in empirical investigation. More specifically, while there are several seemingly authoritative statements made about South Asia and the Caribbean, there is not a single scholarly reference in the long bibliography. In contrast, Sheila Patterson's work (discussed later) which contains a brief bibliography is balanced, drawing on relevant literature on Caribbean history and society. Rex's fiction is underlined, for example, by his claim that West Indian economies were such that migrants from the region could not return and that they left the region at a time when these economies were undergoing further decline. But this is the very opposite to what perhaps the most vigorous generation of Caribbean economists was writing at the time (e.g. Girvan, 1971; Jefferson, 1972), as they outlined what was perhaps the greatest economic boom in the region since the mid-nineteenth century.

Second, the Rexian prophecies wittingly or unwittingly reproduced and gave new life in Britain to past colonial stereotypes that developed from the nineteenth century. This was perhaps particularly strong in the Caribbean, where people of African and South Asian backgrounds met in what was to be conflict situations as the colonial regime threw them into competition. There is perhaps no clearer example of this than Walter

Rodney's (1981) description of the construction of the subservient 'Sammy' (from the venerable 'swamy') and 'Quashie' (from Kwesi). With respect to post-imperial Britain, it is fortunate that the vast majority of people from the Caribbean and Asian communities have not too fervently allowed those social analysts who have a voice within the academic and the policy worlds to influence African-Caribbean and Asian perceptions of each other.

A more nuanced, knowledgeable example of the theme of comparing communities is found in the work of Sheila Patterson (1965). In *Dark strangers: a study of West Indians in London* (first published 1963), Patterson thought that while immigrants from Continental Europe would 'integrate' into British society, West Indians would 'assimilate', but she stressed:

> Predictions in such matters are always dangerous. On the strength of the Brixton material and the history of the past migrant settlements in this country, however, *I would be prepared to hazard the guess that over the next decades in Britain the West Indian migrants and their children will follow in the steps of the Irish;* they will, though not without the checks and reverses inevitable in such processes, become acceptable as a regular and permanent component of the local labour force, gradually raising their living standards and fanning out of the central areas of settlement. An able minority will push upwards into the skilled and professional strata, where a trail has already been blazed by an upper- and middle-class minority who preceded the mass migration from the West Indies. *This adaptation and advancement will lead to closer social relationships with the local population, and probably to increased intermarriage and to an at least partial biological absorption of the West Indians in the local population – as happened in the case of over 10,000 freed coloured slaves in nineteenth-century London, and to many thousands of white ex-soldiers, indentured labourers, and settlers in the West Indian islands themselves.*
>
> (Patterson, 1965: 343–4, emphases added)

Several of Patterson's guesses have found echoes in subsequent work (Ward and Jenkins, 1984; Cross and Entzinger, 1988), and are central to more recent discussions (Berrington, 1996; Owen, 1996; Goulbourne, 1998) that cannot be entered into here.

A cautionary note

Developments since the late 1980s suggest that Sheila Patterson was correct in cautioning about predicting the future; these developments also serve to render much of Rexian sociology of communities in Britain to be false prophesies based on assumptions without either theoretical or empirically/historically verified foundations. Apart from major changes in the wider world, these developments have been punctuated by the Rushdie Affair at the end of the 1980s, the demand for separate schools by faith communities (particularly by Muslims groups), physical conflicts on the streets of northern cities (Bradford, Oldham, etc.) and between Asian and (Rex's) 'native' communities, the growth of post-9/11 Muslim fundamentalisms (as well as Christian variants), growing security fear in public places, and the protest of some Sikhs resulting in a play in Birmingham being taken off the stage in the middle of the first decade of the twenty-first century. The fear that many inner-city authorities had of West Indian youths in the 1970s and 1980s has become a generalised fear of youth characterised by hoodies, those emerging folk-devils. The 1970s and 1980s fears have also given way to a far more frightening culture of violence (particularly over drugs) within Caribbean communities themselves, not so much against Rex's white society. The situation is at once more complex than the prophesy and more hopeful in terms of integration.

Rex's carefully crafted remarks about 'withdrawal', the building of utopias, and so on were central to his expectations of how former colonial immigrants would integrate into British society. It has been seen how, for Rex, Asians exhibited traits of engaging with the majority society, while his West Indians withdraw, become hostile, and develop something Rex described as 'a culture of resistance'. For him this trait is particularly strong in three areas of British life: religion, politics, and mass culture. Developments to the contrary over the last half-century (since the 1960s) have demonstrated how apparently benign and genuine social analysis can come to be seen as nothing more than the uncritical reproduction (and boost of life) of past colonial/imperial prejudices grounded in ideologies of racial and ethnic dominance and hegemony. In terms of the lived lives of people of Caribbean backgrounds in Britain over the last half-century, the question must be asked whether any social commentator can seriously say that their institutions and social practices which initially met with hostility and rejection have not negotiated entries into the mainstream of the extant social order.

To illustrate without labouring the point: the vernacular language of the street, style and apparel, music, sports, Christian forms of worship, and so forth of the majority population as well as other minorities have been indelibly influenced and directed (though not controlled) by Caribbeans. Admittedly, this has been unplanned, and helped by the cultural representations of African-Americans in the Atlantic world. However, we would be hard put to find a single more powerful reason for this than the fact that Caribbeans – of all racio-ethnic backgrounds – have caused an offence to ethno-racial ideologues precisely because the most fundamental values of people from the region have been the following:

- the acceptance of each person as an individual;
- an acceptance of the equality of all groups into which humans have sought to identify themselves;
- a willingness to allow people from other communities into Caribbean Creole communities;
- the absence of sharp and exclusive ethno-racial boundaries and the porous nature of these boundaries;
- practice of an unbounded ethno-racial pragmatism.

These values are not mere abstractions – indeed, these are not to be found verbally articulated in any grand statement anywhere – but are strongly reflected in all kinds of day-to-day social practices: family and kinship memberships; community organisations' membership; religious affiliation; and political participation in political parties espousing conflicting (though not necessarily physically violent) ideologies. It is interesting that the looseness, the absence of hard boundaries, and the rejection of strictly controlled patriarchal social orders have been generally seen as an absence of cultural values or cultural weaknesses.

While individuals and communities from Asian and Caribbean backgrounds have to cope with racism and exclusion in Britain, it cannot be denied that the laws, as evolved in the general majority society, have helped to force social change in the crucial areas of housing, education, employment, and so forth, so that many of the crudities of racist practice prevalent up to the end of the 1980s appear less obvious in the first decade of the new millennium. More significantly, the uniformly constructed entities of racial and ethnic identities that Rex and his contemporaries envisaged leading to an underclass have not materialised; to be sure, elements of all new minority communities have been caught in a cycle of deprivation that sometimes resembles that of the underclass as described in American cities, and some commentators have relied on this as justification of the atrocities in London on 7 July 2005. But the important point is that there has been significant social upward mobility; in the case of Caribbeans this has been accompanied by downward social mobility, but this may be due as much to racist exclusion as to these groups' inability to mobilise their social capital to attain desired ends. In other words, the situation is far more complex than was envisaged, but in this complexity there are more social spaces for desirable change than was predicted.

So, we may very well ask whether the present policy and academic concerns have transcended earlier ones, and whether the research questions have moved alongside what may be happening in the transformation of British society. In terms of approach, there have certainly been some changes. In the first place, there is no longer a comprehensive approach taking into account a wide range of issues such as education, employment, housing, and law and order, and pertaining to a specifically located community and its expected collective life. Instead, with few exceptions, such as Bauman (1996), there have been more piecemeal accounts taking specific aspects of social life about particular groups within larger communities. While there was something of a brief lull of interest in questions about integration, absorption, or assimilation, some major events – pertaining in the main to the lives of Asian/Muslim communities (e.g. the Rushdie Affair; riots in northern cities between 'hosts' and Asian communities; post-9/11 security fears, etc.) – have given new force to such issues, enveloping both policy and academic communities. The research community may have moved away from the 'big picture' to a series of fragmented pictures, with the relationships between each not clear enough to draw general conclusions about the direction of post-imperial British society. But in the wake of atrocities such as the London suicide bombers of Thursday 7 July, there is a tendency to revert too hastily to a notion of community and communal loss that is all too actively destroyed by academic and political commentators who allocate value/worth on the one hand and, on the other, dispense non-value and worthlessness.

The vocabulary and concepts have changed: the possession, access to, and utilisation of 'social capital' have absorbed those of 'networks', 'cultural strengths', 'absence of culture', and so forth. However, are we not in a situation of *'plus ça change, plus c'est la même chose'* (the more things change, the more they remain the same). That is, the change in vocabulary should not be taken to have significantly affected the substantial contents, concerns, and methodological approaches in social policy and academic discourses. If in some quarters of sound social research these methodological limitations have been surmounted, it is still the case that crude and misleading comparisons between individuals, families, and whole communities continue to inform much public debate, media representation, and too much policy research.

Conclusion

But perhaps this is too pessimistic a view of public debates, media coverage, and the academic enterprise. After all, there now appears to be a reluctance to compare different groups in terms of the perceived strengths of one and the perceived weaknesses of the other. Between the census dates 1991 and 2001 there appears to be a more self-critical approach to the study of new minority communities; there has been less of a willingness to see these communities as being fixed and eternally formed groups. However, to arrive at a more critical social studies position that can be of use to both understanding social processes and hopefully informing or influencing social policy, we desperately need to incorporate a heavy dose of intellectual integrity into our perceptions and analyses of the world around us. In doing so, there is no need for the baring or the flagellation of the *angst* soul, but perhaps we could all do no worse than heed Banton's (2005) recent admonition to social analysts to reflect on past mistakes. This might enable us continually to think through ways of moving away from what Weber called our 'demonic' positions, and towards a more balanced comparative methodology in studies of Britain's kaleidoscopic post-imperial society.

References

Banton, M. (2005) 'Finding, and correcting, my mistakes', *Sociology*, 39(3), 463–80.

Baumann, G. (1996) *Contesting culture: discourses of identity in multiethnic London*, Cambridge: Cambridge University Press.

Berrington, A. (1996) 'Marriage patterns and inter-ethnic unions' in D. Coleman and J. Salt (eds) *Ethnicity in the 1991 Census: demographic characteristics of the ethnic minority populations*, vol. 1, London: OPCS.

Bryceson, D. and Vuorela, U. (eds) (2002) *The transnational family: new European frontiers and global networks*, Oxford: Berg.

Cross, M. and Entzinger, H. (eds) (1988) *Lost illusions: Caribbean minorities in Britain and The Netherlands*, London: Routledge.

Dench, G. (1975) *Maltese in London*, London: Routledge and Kegan Paul.

Dench, G. (1986) *Minorities in the open society: prisoners of ambivalence*, London: Routledge and Kegan Paul.

Fryer, P. (1984) *Staying power: the history of Black people in Britain*, London: Pluto.

Furstenberg, F. (2005) 'Neighbours and social capital', unpublished keynote address, *Wither social capital?: international conference on social capital, Families and Social Capital ESRC Research Group*, London South Bank University.

Girvan, N. (1971) *Foreign capital and economic underdevelopment in Jamaica*, Kingston: Institute of Social and Economic Research, University of the West Indies.

Goulbourne, H. (1990) 'The contribution of West Indian groups to British politics' in H. Goulbourne (ed.) *Black politics in Britain*, Aldershot: Avebury.

Goulbourne, H. (1991) *Ethnicity and nationalism in post-imperial Britain*, Cambridge: Cambridge University Press.

Goulbourne, H. (1998) *Race relations in Britain since 1945*, London: Macmillan.

Goulbourne, H. (2002) *Caribbean transnational experience*, London: Pluto Press.

Goulbourne, H. and Chamberlain, M. (eds) (2001) *Caribbean families in Britain and the trans Atlantic world*, London: Macmillan.

Jefferson, O. (1972) *The post-War economic development of Jamaica*, Institute of Social and Economic Research, University of the West Indies.

Jenkins, R. (1967) 'Racial equality in Britain' in A. Lester (ed.) *Essays and speeches by Roy Jenkins*, London: Collins.

Mills, C. Wright (1970) *The sociological imagination*, London: Penguin.

Oakley, R. (1979) 'Family, kinship and patronage: the Cypriot migration to Britain' in S.V. Khan (ed.) *Minority families in Britain: support and stress*, London: Macmillan.

Owen, D. (1996) 'Size, structure and growth of the ethnic minority populations' in D. Coleman and J. Salt (eds) *Ethnicity in the 1991 Census: demographic characteristics of the ethnic minority populations*, vol. 1, London: OPCS.

Parekh, B. (2002) *The future of multi-ethnic Britain: the Parekh Report*, London: The Runnymede Trust.

Patterson, S. (1965) *Dark strangers: a study of West Indians in London*, Harmondsworth: Penguin.

Plummer, K. (2003) *Intimate Citizenship: Private Decisions and Public Dialogues*, London: University of Washington Press.

Rex, J. (1970) *Race relations in sociological theory*. London: Routledge and Kegan Paul.

Rex, J. and Tomlinson, S. (1979) *Colonial immigrants in a British city: a class analysis*. London: Routledge and Kegan Paul.

Rodney, W. (1981) *A history of the Guyanese working people, 1881–1905*, London: Heinemann Educational Books.

Sherwood, M. (1991) 'Race, nationality and employment among Lascar seamen, 1660 to 1945', *New Community*, 17(2).

South London Press, 16 February 2006, pp. 4–5.

Swann, M. (1985) *Education for all: report of the Committee of Inquiry into the education of children from ethnic minority groups*, Cmnd 9453. London: HMSO.

Tonnies, F. (1955) *Community and association*, trans. C. P. Loomis. London: Routledge and Kegan Paul.

Ward, R. and Jenkins, R. (eds) (1984) *Ethnic communities in business: strategies for economic survival*, Cambridge: Cambridge University Press.

Weeks, J., Holland, J. and Waites, M. (eds) (2003) *Sexualities and society: a reader*, Cambridge: Polity.

An earlier version of this chapter was published in (2006) *Community, Work and Family*, 9(3) 235–50. I am grateful to the editors for permission to publish this revised version here.

Chapter 6

Secondary analysis in investigating family change

Exploring substantive and conceptual questions[1]

Val Gillies

Introduction

I begin this chapter with an explanation. To date, my experience of conducting secondary analysis has been in terms of reworking material collected while coworking on specific projects. I have not, as yet, revisited data from a substantially different timeframe to explore social change, but this is not due to lack of commitment or the want of trying. Over the last five years, Rosalind Edwards and I have put together various funding bids aimed at harnessing the value of 50-year-old data in understanding family change. While we have not yet secured a grant that would enable us to put our proposals into action, we have necessarily done a lot of thinking about the issues involved in attempting an historical comparative analysis of qualitative data. It is this thinking that forms the basis of this chapter. More specifically, I document some of the challenges we have faced in constructing a methodologically feasible proposal to investigate social change in parenting. Our aim was to revisit interview studies from the 1960s and compare them with contemporary data but, as I will demonstrate, this is far from a straightforward process. I begin with a brief discussion of some of the current debates around secondary analysis of qualitative data, exploring critiques of the process and their counter critiques. I then outline in more detail the particular research question we are hoping to explore through historical comparison. The rest of the chapter addresses the specific problems and dilemmas we faced in devising a method, as well as the potential for secondary analysis to contribute to understandings of social change.

Secondary analysis: problems and potentials

Interest in secondary analysis of qualitative data has grown significantly over the years. Nevertheless, as an Economic and Social Research Council consultation exercise revealed, it is still something of a controversial practice among the research community (Henwood and Laing 2003). Methodological concerns about the extent to which detailed, situated studies can be re-analysed have been the subject of considerable debate. This is in contrast to secondary analysis of quantitative data, which is well-established and rarely questioned. From a quantitative perspective data exists independently from the researcher and so can be reused in the future to assess the reliability and validity of particular findings, but where qualitative approaches are concerned, interactions between researchers and interviewees are viewed as crucial in shaping interpretations. As a result, the original context in which data is, or was, collected is central to any qualitative analysis. The significance placed on context is often conveyed through reference to the intimate bond that the researcher inevitably develops with the data, particularly when they have designed the framework, immersed themselves in the field, and drawn on personally grounded insights to make interpretations. Martyn Hammersley (1997) has described the 'cultural habitus' that is acquired through direct involvement in fieldwork, and suggests that the key role of this intuitive knowledge and experience limits the usability of other people's data.

This view appears to be reflected in what Paul Thompson (2000: 1) has called the 'strange silence close to the heart of the qualitative research community'. This silence is characterised by a general reluctance to draw on material created by other research teams. Consequently, the notion of data not existing independently from the researcher has been a serious barrier to the development of qualitative secondary analysis (Corti 2000). These concerns extend even towards the practice of researchers involved in the original study later returning to re-analyse their data. This is something Natasha Mauthner, Odette Parry, and Kathryn Backett Milburn (1998) have discussed in some detail. They have drawn attention to the way memories fade and personal perspectives change over time, and have argued that this drastically alters the researchers' relationship to the original data. From this perspective qualitative data is integrally formed by the conditions it is created in, and these conditions can not be archived for future reuse. In other words, while the positivist conditions of quantitative data collection are highly compatible with reuse, qualitative research is context specific. Mauthner and colleagues are particularly critical of the idea that this problem of context can be overcome simply by archiving more background information alongside the original studies. They dismiss the implication that this can repair or complete the data set, and argue that these practical attempts to hold on to the contextual substance of qualitative research mask more fundamental epistemological questions. As they explain:

> Issues surrounding the complexities of returning to old datasets arose for us upon revisiting our own data, collected in previously completed research projects, for the purposes of generating new theories and findings. Most of our difficulties arose because we realised that our data were a product of the dynamic, dialectical and reflexive nature of

a particular research encounter which both described but also delim-
ited the meaning of the data.

(Mauthner et al. 1998: 736)

However, those advocating secondary analysis have engaged extensively
with these critiques and have begun to construct a robust defence. For example, Louise Corti (2000) and others (Corti and Thompson 2004; Heaton
2004) have pointed out, that reuse of data is actually an extremely common
practice, given that research teams often share material and that researchers
are regularly employed just to conduct interviews. Niamh Moore highlights
just how blurred the boundaries are between primary and secondary
research. She poses a chicken or egg question, asking what comes first, secondary analysis or secondary data. More specifically, she argues that
secondary analysis is not analysis of pre-existing data, but instead involves a
re-contextualisation of data.

> Once the data is transformed through the process of re-contextualisa-
> tion, it is not so much that we now have a new entity to be termed
> 'secondary data' and which might require a new methodology to be
> termed secondary analysis, rather, that through the re-contextualisa-
> tion, the order of the data has been transformed, thus secondary
> analysis is perhaps more usefully rendered as primary analysis of a dif-
> ferent order of data.

(Moore 2005: 9)

Moore also criticises the tendency to evaluate the potential of qualitative
secondary analysis on the same basic terms as quantitative reuse. For example, Mauthner and colleagues apply a quantitative framework of data reuse
to argue that qualitative data is different and therefore not amenable to secondary analysis. However, as Moore points out, there are other points of
comparison that may yield more useful insights, such as documentary
analysis and oral history.

Another important point, made by Mike Savage, is that no form of data
– qualitative or quantitative – is ever neutral. Context is just as important in
the construction of quantitative data, but the major difference is that this is
made transparent and is built into qualitative methodology. As he states:

> But here we can see a real advantage for the secondary analysis of qual-
> itative data in that the research process is less easily written out of the
> archived data than is the case for survey sources, where subsequent
> researchers usually just have access to the codebook and the data set.
> For these quantitative sources, the abstraction process is often so com-
> plete that the traces of the original fieldwork have been altogether
> covered over. This process of covering over the traces of the fieldwork is

much more difficult for qualitative research, and this is a fact which should be celebrated, rather than seen as a 'problem' (as it might be from within a positivist perspective).

(Savage 2005: 43)

It seems that in the face of longstanding concerns and critiques a relatively strong case can be made for the validity of reusing qualitative data. But significant methodological questions remain, and these become more complex when qualitative data reuse is proposed as part of a comparative historical analysis. As I will demonstrate, attempts to compare data sets across different time frames raise many more questions about commensurability.

The broader context: understandings of change and family

As I explained in the introduction, this paper derives from an attempt to put together a research proposal to explore family change. Before I can discuss the specific methodological problems we encountered, I need to set the context framing the research in terms of sociological understandings of change and family. At a broad level, it is important to recognise that sociologists have a particular preoccupation with the nature and impact of social change (Abercrombie and Warde 1992; Berman 1983). The discipline itself was founded as an attempt to theorise the impact of emerging structural changes, and the theme of transformation can be traced from a focus on nineteenth-century industrial versus pre-industrial societies, to a more contemporary interest in the individualising effects of post-industrialisation (Stanley 1992). But this fixation on change has been criticised on a number of levels. It has been pointed out that social change is sometimes viewed as a necessary condition for study, and that sociologists often tend to structure their research questions around the experience of change (Abercrombie and Warde 1992). This focus on transformation may be at the expense of equally significant social continuities, thereby obscuring, or even distorting, enduring aspects of social life.

For the most part, evidence of change comes from large-scale quantitative surveys like the census or the General Household Survey in the UK. This data has been used to back up transformation theories which stand independently from more grounded empirical research. For example, the pronouncements of macro, demographic change made by major sociological theorists like Ulrich Beck and Elizabeth Beck-Gernsheim (1995, 1998, 2002) and Anthony Giddens (1991) are not based on research-led explorations of lives as they are actually lived. Yet empirical research is vital to assess the real significance of change. A reliance on abstract and quantitative data risks overstating the meaning or effect of observable changes. For example, we can reliably state that less people get married today than was the case 50 years ago, but we can be less confident in interpreting the real meaning of this for people's lives. Qualitative research continues to point to the enduring significance of family and family lives (Ribbens McCarthy *et al.* 2003; Williams 2004).

It has also been pointed out that interpretations of social change are never theoretically or ideologically neutral, with disputes continuing to rage about the definitions and significance of change (Abercrombie and Warde 1992; Crow 2002), particularly in relation to families. Many writers have doubted the basis on which assumptions of social change are often made, with some questioning the way a fixed 'Othered' past is defined and differentiated from an ephemeral present (Adam 1996). There are also questions raised about the possibility of mistaking of cyclical patterns for linear transformation (Stanley 1992). In response to these debates, researchers have begun to adopt a more in-depth empirical approach to social change. Some have conducted comparative re-studies based on classic works from the 1950s by Clive Rosser and Chris Harris (Aull Davies and Charles 2002; Chapter 8 this volume), and Michael Young and Peter Willmott (Phillipson 2001; Chapter 8 this volume). While these re-studies provide a valuable insight into the nature and meaning of change, they stop short of re-analysing the original data. Yet sociological frameworks themselves change over time and this can make distinct social transformations harder to detect without re-analysis.

The concept of social change may be formative in sociology as a discipline but it is particularly central to contemporary theorising on family and community life. It is this specific context that has stimulated our interest in conducting an historical comparison. Debates in this field tend to be structured around the premise that social and economic changes have profoundly influenced the way people relate to each other in family and intimate life (Gillies 2003). From one perspective, post-industrialisation has led to a de-traditionalisation and individualisation of social life, associated with rising rates of divorce, cohabitation, and births outside of marriage. This is viewed as a 'breakdown' of established social ties leading to the disintegration of moral frameworks. Family relationships are seen in terms of a fracturing of traditional support systems and a decline in values of duty and responsibility. From this perspective great strain is being placed on the institution of the family, drastically undermining the practice of good parenting and damaging social cohesion more generally (Coleman 1990; Davies 1993; Dennis and Erdos 1992; Etzioni 1993; Fevre 2000; Murray 1994).

Concerns over this feared demise in community relations and trust have generated an interest in social capital as a framework for theorising and promoting social resources. The works of Robert Putnam (1993, 1995, 1996) and James Coleman (1988, 1990, 1991) in the field have been particularly influential. Both theorists identify diminishing levels of social capital, linking this to changes in parenting and family life in what Rosalind Edwards has termed a 'social capital lost story' (Edwards 2004). But other theorists take a more optimistic view of social change. They emphasise a greater diversity and plurality of lifestyles, arguing this generates new opportunities for more democratic family relations. They see this as augmenting rather than diminishing the resources that parents can draw on for support. So from this perspective people are now seeking more fulfilling family and community relationships. These are based on egalitarian values of respect and negotiation, as opposed to duty and obligation. This is seen as hailing a 'new golden age' of social capital. Trends towards cohabitation, separation, and re-partnership are viewed as indicators of a shift in family relations, moving from a 'community of need' to 'elective affinities' (Beck-Gernsheim 1998). Parents can now build their own social networks, seeking out and accessing support and knowledge for themselves. New 'families of choice' are said to be emerging from a context of diverse social interactions, marking the generation of alternative social capital networks and parenting resources (Beck and Beck-Gernsheim 1995, 2002; Beck-Gernsheim 1998, 2002; Giddens 1991; Stacey 1996; Weeks 1995; Weeks *et al.* 2001).

In contrast to arguments of demise or regeneration in family and community life, there is also a perspective that questions the extent of social change. This point of view cites studies which emphasise the importance individuals continue to place on family relationships and obligations (Jamieson 1998; Gillies *et al.* 2001; Ribbens McCarthy *et al.* 2003). It is suggested that while analysis of current trends in family forms and household composition can emphasise increased diversity in living arrangements, these figures also reveal an enduring continuity of traditional ties with the majority of families still composed of heterosexual couples and their biological children. In addition, some theorists have claimed that diversity and plurality has always been a feature of family relationships. For example, Graham Crow (2002; Chapter 2 this volume) suggests there may have been considerably more fluidity and diversity in past family relationships than was previously recognised, while Liz Stanley (1992) draws on her own qualitative research to show how official, abstract definitions of family structure and employment status can conceal considerable ambiguity and complexity. Similarly, the emphasis placed on change is challenged by the theorist Pierre Bourdieu's (1986, 1990) view of social capital as inextricably linked to a number of other central resources. These other capitals are seen by Bourdieu as determining an individual's standing as well as their likely trajectory. So from this perspective contemporary society is witnessing neither the decline nor the transformation of social capital. Instead we are seeing its consistent deployment in the reproduction of privilege and inequality. Despite these differing views on the significance of change in family life, the social capital lost story appears to be the most influential at the moment.

This view has underpinned a number of recent social policy initiatives designed to tackle the effects of family change by regulating childrearing practices in Britain. Premised on an assumption of the breakdown of social relationships and a loss of collective social norms, recent years have seen an explicit focus on parenting as a designated area of policy intervention. A raft of initiatives has been set up including the National Family and Parenting Institute, Parentline Plus, the Sure Start programme, and the Parenting Fund. Underlying these policies are assumptions about the deteriorating nature of contemporary family relationships and support systems. This preoccupation with transformation is also reflected in the attention given to the concept of social capital in policy, through a focus on bolstering community and the resources and support that are generated from social networks (e.g. ONS 2001, and commentaries in Baron *et al.* 2000; Gamarnikow and Green 1999).

Comparative analysis: addressing conceptual problems

It was against the backdrop of this policy concern with parenting that our contemporary study of parenting resources was conducted (Edwards and Gillies 2005). The project was called 'Resources in Parenting: Access to Capitals' and it was made up of two phases. The first phase was based on an extensive survey of parents' public norms around support, while the second phase was based on theoretically sampled qualitative interviews to examine everyday practices. In line with Bourdieu's work, we found that the resources or 'capitals' accessible to parents were inextricably linked in terms of economic, cultural and social resources. We also found that parents in our sample were generally not isolated or unsure about who to turn to for support (Edwards and Gillies 2005). In short, we found very little evidence to suggest there had been substantial decline in social capital, but we had no baseline to consider this in terms of change or continuity. Identifying and theorising change within the context of this debate deserves a more concerted effort, particularly given the significance it is accorded within the field of sociology and theories of family and parenting.

Qualitative, empirical research tends to expose the contradictory, tangled complexity of real life experience, often standing in stark contrast to neatly packaged theoretical accounts of social change. According to Graham Crow (2002; Chapter 2 this volume), sociological community studies were (and remain) particularly effective empirical tools for evaluating abstract theorising on the nature of social change. He suggests they represent a grounded analysis of social relationships as they are lived in a locality. The data exists as crucial temporal evidence in the face of evolving conceptual and methodological expectations. More specifically, in our view, the existence of archived in-depth community and family studies from the 1960s represents a valuable source material for the study of family and social change. This period is often identified in both 'social capital lost' and 'new golden age' perspectives as the historical point after which either decline or renewal began to take hold. Re-analysis of this early data offers an opportunity to capitalise on the situated details of everyday life. It would allow us to engage with theories of social transformation in a more critical and systematic way. More specifically, the data would potentially enable us to compare parenting resources and social networks across time to assess claims of social change. This was our major aim in drawing up a research bid, and we designed a project that would answer the following questions:

- Has the experience of parenting children changed significantly over the last 40 years? What differences and continuities can be identified?
- Have the resources and social support networks available to particular groups of parents diminished, modified, or remained relatively consistent over time?
- What is the relationship between change and continuity across different time frames? How can social change be understood in terms of family life and parenting?
- How appropriate are current family policy initiatives? To what extent is their emphasis on change and social fragmentation justified?

However, any attempt to pinpoint social change involves trying to under-stand the past from the viewpoint of the present. This entails addressing intricate conceptual complexities, making exploring social change through secondary analysis about much more than a simple historical comparison of data. One problem to be faced is the shifting nature of sociological interest. The focus of research evolves over time and this limits the contex-tual commensurability between different historically and culturally specific data sets. This generates numerous conceptual and methodological ques-tions, and is something that researchers conducting re-studies also encounter. Charlotte Aull Davies and Nickie Charles (2002) have discussed this in relation to their major comparative re-study based on Rosser and Harris's (1965) classic work *The Family and Social Change* (see also Chapter 8 this volume). They became aware of inevitable discontinuities between their source data from the 1960s and the contemporary material they collected. This required them to deviate slightly from the original research design. In this re-study, evolving understandings of ethnographic research required consideration and compromise in terms of methods and methodology. These considerations would also apply if we were to conduct a secondary analysis of historically situated data to explore social change in parenting. Comparisons across different time frames will inevitably encounter substantive and conceptual gaps. These gaps are immediately apparent when an attempt is made to match current research data with past studies. Rather than replicating a previous study, we are starting with current research and aiming to conduct a reconstructive re-analysis of rele-vant past studies. Our contemporary marker for conducting a comparative secondary analysis would be the in-depth interviews with mothers and fathers that were collected as part of parenting resources study. But while this contemporary research shares many of the same themes of earlier community studies, it diverges sharply in terms of focus and theory, as Table 6.1 below demonstrates.

As I have outlined, parenting is a current concern in the UK, and this reflects a policy-driven preoccupation with parenting support. Although there is a long history of evaluative, quantitative research on parenting practice, few qualitative studies based on parents' own accounts were conducted in the past. Those that were carried out predominantly concerned themselves with aspects of development and parent–child interaction. As a result, finding historical comparative data to contextualise claims about the decline of social capital is not just a matter of returning to similar, earlier research; equivalent studies simply do not exist. Instead, relevant themes and accounts are embedded within a range of topic areas that were the concerns of their day. For example, the themes of community and class dominated the sociological agenda in the 1960s.

While these studies should still provide useful markers for comparison, further complications arise from their characteristic focus on specific populations. The classic community studies inevitably centre on social relations in particular geographical areas. Many early studies of social class are similarly place-based in order to explore demographic shifts, such as the establishment of new towns or the influx of the middle class into working-class areas. In contrast, our contemporary data on parenting resources is geographically dispersed throughout England and Scotland, so it is not possible to make any area-specific comparison. Nevertheless, it could be argued that a simple place-based analysis would risk confounding short-term or area-specific demographic change with more general concepts of social transformation. For example, Bethnal Green in East London is the site of the classic Young and Willmott study. Although 50 years later an attempt has been made to replicate this research by Dench et al. (2006), the area has been transformed by new patterns of immigration, making any such place-based analysis very specific to Bethnal Green. Consequently it could be argued that the range of environments which make up our contemporary sample constitute a more rigorous starting point to explore change and continuity.

Table 6.1 Shifting social contexts: discontinuities in data sets

Past data	Contemporary data
Preoccupation with community and class	Preoccupation with parenting support
Place-based community studies	Geographically dispersed
Focus on particular social characteristics, e.g. working-class communities or single mothers	Focus on a range of social characteristics

Early sociological studies were not just place-based. They were also confined to specific social categories like class, gender, or family structure. For example, some studies focused exclusively on working-class communities, on wives/mothers, or on single mothers. In this case, achieving a meaningful historical comparison would involve disembedding appropriate data from a range of sources. Fortunately, the ESDS Qualidata archive at Essex University has preserved a number of classic studies conducted in the 1950s, 1960s, and 1970s. During an initial visit to the archive we were able to identify a number of data sets with the potential to provide historical benchmarks for our comparative analysis of parenting.

The Affluent Worker Collection: Goldthorpe and colleagues conducted semi-structured interviews in the early 1960s with male factory workers from Luton and Cambridge and their wives, exploring the themes of class, community, parent–child relations, family life, education, friends, household budgets, social life, social change, and social mobility. Eight hundred and forty-seven survey questionnaires, handwritten interview transcripts, notes, and other materials are available for re-analysis.

Salford Slum Re-housing Study: Marsden conducted in-depth interviews in the early 1960s, exploring the impact of re-housing on working-class families. The themes of kinship, household organisation, children's education, and local neighbourhood are explored. One hundred typed transcripts are available for re-analysis along with written field notes and other supporting material.

Parents and Education: Marsden conducted in-depth interviews in the early 1960s with a wide range of parents to investigate parental choices in education, and the influence they exert over the children's schooling. One hundred and forty-three, mostly handwritten, transcripts are available for re-analysis, with written notes and supporting material.

Mothers Alone: Poverty and the Fatherless Family: Marsden conducted in-depth interviews with lone mothers in the mid-1960s, exploring the experience of parenting alone. One hundred and sixteen typewritten interview transcripts, along with written notes and other supporting material, have been digitised and are available online as part of the Qualidata archive.

Early data on parenting resources and family is embedded in a range of these themes and topic areas. In fact it could be argued that orthodox theories of social capital have merely reframed these concerns, leading to a differently termed focus on social exclusion/inclusion, parenting values, and support. As Mildred Blaxter (2004) has noted, historically specific understandings of social problems define research frameworks, and as such, studies are embedded in social trends which may themselves be representative of social change.

Further complexity is introduced when we consider the changing analytical contexts governing research agendas. Context is an intractable obstacle to the simple measurement of historically situated data sets, but it can be argued that re-analysis of past data from a contemporary frame of reference has the potential to change our understanding of the present by generating new perspectives on the past. Previous traditions of theory and inquiry may have limited understanding of the (now) classic data from contemporary perspectives and concerns (Bornat 2005; Charles 2005; Savage 2005, Chapters 7 and 8 this volume). As Simon Szreter notes, contemporary debates about social and economic change are commonly prone to a view of the past that is 'distorted by hindsight and unwitting present-centredness' (Szreter 2005: 1). As a result, policymakers may initiate or 'reinvent' policies either without reference to the past or without understanding whether, how far, and in what ways the social context has changed (Alcock 2005; Goulbourne 2006). As Martyn Hammersley notes '[t]he past can set us new problems, or cast old problems in a new light' (1997: 135).

The challenge of historically specific research frameworks

In reflecting on re-study methodology, Charlotte Aull Davies and Nikki Charles (2002; Chapter 8 this volume) cite changes in the way class, gender, and ethnicity are now conceptualised. They refer in particular to the distinct, historically specific framework governing early interview schedules. For example, social class definitions were derived from cultural markers with limited contemporary relevance since they tended to be based solely on male 'head of households'. Also, certain questions were deemed to be gender-specific at the time of the original study, and were only asked either of men or of women. Understandings of ethnicity were similarly time-specific, reflecting the predominantly white make-up of the original studies.

Issues around original social class definitions are less significant in conducting a secondary analysis because a new analytical interpretation of class can be overlain on the original study. It is much more problematic if the secondary analysis reveals that different questions were asked of working- and middle-class families in the 1950s and 1960s. In the case of gender, we would expect this divergent focus in early studies of mothers and fathers. Meanings of fatherhood have changed dramatically over the last 50 years (Burghes et al. 1997) and this inevitably shapes the type of data collected at different points in time. But to pursue any analysis of social change, these evolving conceptual frameworks need critical evaluation as points of reference in themselves. There is a tendency to view current approaches to social categories as enlightened in comparison with the 'politically incorrect' assumptions made in the past. Yet contemporary analytic contexts could be viewed as similarly constraining in that they project and promote an ethos of equality in the face of continuing difference and disparity. For example, in our contemporary research on parenting, mothers and fathers were asked exactly the same questions, but this reflects an ideological shift rather than a practical change in gender roles. This was very clear from the interviews themselves which revealed the primary role mothers still play in childrearing.

In discussing their re-study, Aull Davies and Charles (2002; Chapter 8 this volume) also note how the social and practical circumstances of their present day sample differed from their predecessors. The circumstances differed in terms of ethnicity and employment opportunities particularly, although changes may turn out to be place-specific rather than universal. While the minority ethnic make-up of the population as a whole has grown substantially, many areas have remained predominantly white. Others (like Bethnal Green) have seen particular ethnic populations settle. In the case of employment, levels vary from area to area. For example, there are high levels of unemployment in locations affected by the demise of the manufacturing industry (Craig 2003). In terms of our aim to conduct a secondary analysis to explore family change, the most pervasive and widespread employment trend is the mass movement of women into the labour market. Of course there have also been other more concrete changes such as developments in technology (including the availability of computers, mobile phones, cars, washing machines, and other domestic products). We know that change is inevitable to some extent, but the proliferation of different household and family forms should not be taken as a self-evident marker of social transformation. A rigid focus on the structure and definitions of family might belie personal meanings, experiences, and practices, and it may well be that normative typologies conceal far more than they illuminate. An historical comparative analysis of parenting would provide a nuanced insight into how these changes are actually lived.

Yet any secondary analysis of historically located data is likely to be severely constrained by the narrow definitions that were at one time (and sometimes still are) applied to families. Previous studies were confined in the main to married, two-parent, heterosexual couples. Clearly contemporary research findings are just as context-bound. Some barriers to historical comparison (like the expansion in family typologies) might be read as evident of change in themselves, but their impact on people's lives has only been assessed from a perspective in which demographic change is conflated with personal experience. Family life is assumed to be different because statistics suggest change has occurred, but a question remains as to whether these structural changes obscure enduring continuities in the way people actually live and interact with each other.

One way of exploring this question in more depth might be to try and access wider material from oral histories. This approach might work to problematise overly simplistic accounts of cohesive traditional versus fragmented contemporary family forms. It is feasible that in the wealth of archived material that exists there might be evidence for more variability in the actual practice of family than the demographic statistics suggest. In our efforts to design a proposal to conduct an historical comparison we have attempted to factor this in this additional source. The classic community studies could be supplemented, for example, with material from the

Millennium Memory Bank at the British Library. This consists of approximately 6,000 life history interviews collected from a variety of people across Great Britain at the turn of the millennium. Including this material would enable us to explore the extra dimension of 're-membering' experiences of family and parenting from a contemporary reference point.

Addressing practical and ethical issues

Edwards and I set out to design an approach to our own re-analysis that would allow us to work within the limitations and affordances I have outlined. This meant we had to make various decisions concerning the status we accord to the data, sampling rationales, and analytical frameworks. But constructing our research framework was further complicated by the practical implications of dealing with *elderly data*. The advent of word processing and availability of compact, efficient tape recorders have transformed the way qualitative data is collected. In the 1960s, transcripts and notes were predominantly handwritten, although some of these were then typed up manually. Tape recordings, where they were made, have rarely survived. Although Qualidata is currently in the process of categorising and digitalising this original data, it is inevitably a long-term project. While we are able to identify a number of potential sources for historical comparison, the most relevant archived studies are, with the exception of the 'Mothers Alone' collection at the time of writing, still paper-based. They consist of large, typed, and sometimes barely legible handwritten data sets, with no details provided about interviewee characteristics. As a result, identifying and selecting appropriate transcripts would be a labour-intensive and time-consuming process that would likely equal the time and effort involved in primary data collection.

In considering a potential sample framework we realised that efforts to match contemporary and historical sample characteristics exactly may be impossible, or even counterproductive. For example, the sharp rise in numbers of full-time employed mothers means they are unlikely to be a well-represented category in early studies. There is a clear need to contextualise the data before a sampling frame can be constructed, and this amounts to an initial level of analysis. We would need to assess the relevant archived collections by categorising their contents and logging demographic details of interviewees. Then in terms of generating a sample we would need to remain sensitive to the possibility that certain characteristics may themselves constitute a marker of social change. Once a sample for the historical comparison had been identified, we would then need to deal with the socially embedded nature of particular research accounts. We would argue that meaning is made rather than found. From this perspective any historical comparison needs to include an analysis of the original material as a socially produced and socially situated construction. This involves careful analysis of the original researchers' questions, fieldnotes, letters, memos, reports, publications, and any other sources of information. Where possible, consultation with original researchers would also generate crucial background information. This attention to context is not about attempting to fill 'gaps' in the data, as Mauthner and colleagues might view it (1998); it is about illuminating the very particular perspectives knowledge was (and is) created from.

In addition, a number of ethical decisions require careful thought. Confidentiality and consent are of particular concern when dealing with qualitative accounts of family life. ESDS Qualidata presides over a number of procedures to protect the confidentiality of interviewees who have contributed to their collections. Some of these measures include the anonymisation of datasets and the issuing of user undertakings to guard against the dissemination of identifying information. But while it is relatively simple to avoid actual personal names and geographical places, other aspects of an individual's life (such as an unusual job or experience) may be conspicuous. Also, certain identifying details like the names of towns or particular employers can sometimes provide a crucial context when presenting an analysis. The use of interviews from the 1960s neutralises the issue to a certain extent in that data this old often bears little connection to people's current lives. In practice though, there is a need to maintain a balance between including rich, informative detail and disclosing information that might break original promises of privacy and anonymity. However, it should be kept in mind that these kinds of dilemmas are not specific to secondary analysis since all qualitative researchers also face them.

Questions have also been raised as to whether renewed consent should be sought when conducting secondary analysis. While early sociological researchers obtained consent to conduct and disseminate the original research, it is unlikely they gained explicit consent for future reuse. In our case it would be extremely time-consuming or impossible to trace those who were interviewed in the 1960s and get their explicit consent. In fact, this could be viewed as unethical in itself, given that interviewees were often told that no further contact would be made. Again, it could be argued that time renders the information in the research material progressively less relevant to participants themselves. Nevertheless, ethical issues in relation to data reuse remain a serious concern for qualitative researchers. This has been highlighted in an article by Odette Parry and Natasha Mauthner (2004) which draws out the huge complexities around copyright, consent, and confidentiality in relation to qualitative secondary analysis. In response, we would argue that this underlines the extent to which such ethical dilemmas are situation specific and not amenable to universal prescriptions.

Conclusion

This paper represents a plan towards an historical comparative analysis of resources in parenting. I have outlined our own attempts to grapple with epistemological and methodological problems associated with the reuse of contextually embedded qualitative data. We have carefully deliberated on these issues to construct a research design that attempts to work within the constraints discussed in this chapter. Our aim is not to devise a rigid positivist model of historical comparison. We do not suggest that any objective measurement of social change is possible, but we do believe that re-reflecting on markers of the past and the present through a common contemporary lens can broaden understandings – even if the result is to foreground the complexity of distinguishing then from now. As I have stated, we have not yet had the opportunity to put our research proposal into practice, and we are very aware that many more practical and conceptual problems are likely to emerge in the process of actually conducting the analysis. The complex challenges associated with secondary analysis, combined with the shortage of empirical models exploring methods and practices, may partly explain its current under use as a method. This does not detract from its potential to generate crucial new perspectives on the nature and meaning of social change.

Notes

1 This chapters draws heavily on an article published in 2005 with R. Edwards: 'Secondary analysis in exploring family and social change: addressing the issue of context', *Forum: Qualitative Research* 6(1) Art. 44: http:www.qualitative-research.net/fqs-texte/1-05/05-1-44-e.htm.

References

Abercrombie, N. and Warde, A. (eds) (1992) *Social Change in Contemporary Britain*, Cambridge: Polity.

Adam, B. (1996) 'Detraditionalization and the certainty of uncertain futures' in P. Heelas, S. Lash and P. Morris (eds), *Detraditionalization: Critical Reflections on Authority and Identity*, Oxford: Blackwell.

Alcock, P. (2005) 'Maximum feasible understanding – lessons from previous wars on poverty', *Social Policy and Society*, 4(3): 321–30.

Aull Davies, C. and Charles, N. (2002). 'Piano in the parlour: methodological issues in the conduct of a restudy', *Sociological Research Online*, 7(2), http://www.socres online.org.uk/7/2/davies.html.

Baron, S., Field, J. and Schuller, T. (eds) (2000) *Social Capital: Critical Perspectives*, Oxford: Oxford University Press.

Beck, U. and Beck-Gernsheim, E. (1995) *The Normal Chaos of Love*, Cambridge: Polity Press.

Beck, U. and Beck-Gernsheim, E. (2002) *Individualization*, London: Sage.

Beck-Gernsheim, E. (1998) 'On the way to a post-familiar family: from a community of need to elective affinities', *Theory, Culture and Society*, 15(3–4), 53–70.

Beck-Gernsheim, E. (2002) *Re-inventing the Family: In Search of New Lifestyles*, Cambridge: Polity.

Berman, M. (1983) *All That is Solid Melts Into Air*, London: Verso.

Blaxter, M. (2004) 'Understanding health inequalities: from transmitted deprivation to social capital', *International Journal of Social Research Methodology: Theory and Practice*, 7(1), 55–9.

Bornat, J. (18 November 2005) 'Recycling the evidence: different approaches to the reanalysis of gerontological data', *Family, Community and Social Change*, ESRC Seminar 3, London: London South Bank University.

Bourdieu, P. (1986) 'The forms of capital' in J.E. Richardson (ed.), *Handbook of Theory for Researching the Sociology of Education*, Westport. CT: Greenwood Press.

Bourdieu, P. (1990) *The Logic of Practice*, Cambridge: Polity.

Burghes, L., Clarke, L. and Cronin, N. (1997) *Fathers and Fatherhood in Britain*, London: Family Policy Studies Centre.

Charles, N. (28 July 2005) 'The family and social change revisited', *Family, Community and Social Change*, ESRC Seminar 3, London South Bank University.

Coleman, J.S. (1988) 'Social capital in the creation of human capital', *American Journal of Sociology*, 94, 121–53.

Coleman, J.S. (1990) *Foundations of Social Theory*, London: Harvard University Press.

Coleman, J. (1991) 'Prologue: constructed social organisation', in P. Bourdieu and J. Coleman (eds) *Social Theory for a Changing Society*, Oxford: Westview Press.

Corti, L. (2000) 'Progress and problems of preserving and providing access to qualitative data for social research—the international picture of an emerging culture', *Forum: Qualitative Social Research*, 1(3), Art. 2, http://www.qualitative-research.net/fqs-texte/3-00/3-00corti-e.htm.

Corti, L. and Thompson, P. (2004) 'Secondary analysis of archive data' in C. Searle, G. Gobo, J.F. Gubrium and D. Silverman (eds), *Qualitative Research Practice*, London: Sage.

Craig, L. (2003) 'A century of labour market change', *Labour Market Trends*, http://findarticles.com/p/articles/mi_qa3999/is_200303/ai_n9185531 (accessed 3/8/07)

Crow, G. (2002) *Social Solidarities: Theories, Identities and Social Change*, Buckingham: Open University Press.

Davies, J. (1993) *The Family, is it Just Another Lifestyle Choice?*, London: Institute For Economic Affairs.

Dench, G., Gavron, K. and Young, M. (2006) *The New East End: Kinship, Race and Conflict*, London: Profile Books.

Dennis, N. and Erdos, G. (1992) *Families Without Fatherhood*, London: Institute For Economic Affairs.

Edwards, R. (2004) 'Present and absent in troubling ways: families and social capital debates', *The Sociological Review*, 52(1), 1–21.

Edwards, R. and Gillies, V. (2005) *Resources in Parenting: Access to Capitals Project Report*, Families and Social Capital ESRC Research Report 14, London: London South Bank University.

Etzioni, A. (1993) *The Parenting Deficit*, London: Demos.

Fevre, R. (2000) *The Demoralisation of Western Culture*, London: Continuum.

Gamarnikow, E. and Green, A. (1999) 'The third way and social capital: education action zones and a new agenda for education, parents and community?', *International Studies in Sociology of Education*, 9(1), 3–22.

Giddens, A. (1991) *Modernity and Self-identity: Self and Society in the Late Modern Age*, Cambridge: Polity Press.

Gillies, V. (2003) *Family and Intimate Relations: a review of the sociological research*, Families and Social Capital ESRC Research Group Working Paper 2, London: London South Bank University.

Gillies, V., Ribbens McCarthy, J. and Holland, J. (2001) *Pulling Together, Pulling Apart: The Family Lives of Young People*, London: Family Policy Studies Centre and Joseph Rowntree Foundation.

Goulbourne, H. (2006) 'Families, communities and social capital', *Community, Work and Family* 9(3), 235–50.

Hammersley, M. (1997) 'Qualitative data archiving: some reflections on its prospects and problems', *Sociology*, 31(1), 131–42.

Heaton, J. (2004) *Reworking Qualitative Data*, London: Sage.

Henwood, K. and Laing, I. (2003) *Qualitative Research Resources: A Consultation Exercise with UK Social Scientists*, ESRC research report, www.esrcsocietytoday. ac.uk/ESRCInfoCentre/Images/QUADS_ConsultationExercise_tcm6–8010.doc (accessed 3/4/07).

Jamieson, L. (1998) *Intimacy*, Cambridge: Polity Press.

Mauthner, N., Parry, O. and Backett Milburn, K. (1998) 'The data are out there, or are they? Implications for archiving and revisiting qualitative data', *Sociology*, 32(4), 733–45.

Murray, C. (1994) *Underclass: The Crisis Deepens*, London: Institute for Economic Affairs.

Niamh, M. (2005) *(Re)using Qualitative Data?* Paper presented at Methods Workshop: *Qualitative Research Laboratory 'Re-using Qualitative Data'* 28 September, University of Manchester, unpublished.

Parry, O. and Mauthner, N. (2004) 'Whose data are they anyway? Practical, legal and ethical issues in archiving qualitative research data', *Sociology*, 38(1), 139–52.

Phillipson, C. (2001) 'The family and community life of older people: social networks and social support in three urban areas', *Ageing and Society*, 18(3), 259–89.

Putnam, R. (1993) *Making Democracy Work: Civic Traditions in Modern Italy*, Princeton: Princeton University.

Putnam, R. (1995) 'Bowling alone: America's declining social capital', *Journal of Democracy*, 6(1), 65–78.

Putnam, R. (1996) 'The strange disappearance of civic America', *Policy*, Autumn, 3–15.

Ribbens McCarthy, J., Edwards, R. and Gillies, V. (2003) *Making Families: Moral Tales of Parenting and Step-parenting*, York: Sociology Press.

Savage, M. (2005) 'Revisiting classic qualitative studies', *Forum: Qualitative Social Research* [Online Journal], 6(1), Art. 31. http://www.qualitative-research.net/fqs-texte/1–05/05–1-31-e.htm.

Stacey, J. (1996) *In the Name of the Family: Rethinking Family Values in the Postmodern Age*, Boston: Beacon Press.

Stanley, L. (1992) 'Changing households, changing work' in N. Abercrombie and A. Warde (eds), *Social Change in Contemporary Britain*, Cambridge: Polity.

Szreter, S. (2005) *Health and Wealth, History and Policy*, http://www.historyandpolicy.org/archive/policy-paper-34.html (accessed 3/8/07).

Thompson, P. (2000) 'Re-using qualitative research data: a personal account', *Forum: Qualitative Social Research*, 1(3), Art. 27, http://www.qualitative-research.net/fqs-texte/3–00/3–00thompson-e.htm.

Weeks, J. (1995) *Inventing Moralities: Sexual Values in an Age of Uncertainty*, New York: Columbia University Press.

Weeks, J., Donovan, C. and Heaphy, B. (2001) *Same Sex Intimacies: Families of Choice and Other Life Experiments*, London: Routledge.

Williams, F. (2004) *Rethinking Families*, London: Calouste Gulbenkian Foundation.

Chapter 7

Recycling the evidence

Different approaches to the re-analysis of elite life histories

Joanna Bornat and Gail Wilson

Introduction

In this chapter we consider the re-analysis of one very specific body of data: the life histories of a select group of pioneers of geriatric medicine from the point of view of what they tell us about the changing attitudes to family and community of one group of professionals. The original data were collected in 1991 in the form of life history interviews by Professor Margot Jefferys and two co-researchers. Her purpose was to present the story, in their own words, of the men (predominantly) who founded the geriatric specialty in mid-twentieth century. As she explains, they were contesting:

> The predominant view, one shared by the public as well as the majority of the medical profession – most of whom would have been trained in the high prestige voluntary hospitals – ... that sickness in old age could not be cured or treated.
>
> (Jefferys 2000: 76)

The interviewees were selected for their role and pre-eminence in this field, and the stories they tell are moral as well as professional accounts of career development (Bornat, 2004). Margot Jefferys elaborates: 'In telling their stories, many of our interviewees were recalling their own awakening as well as a life of professional campaigning against inequality and exclusion in health care provision' (Jefferys 2000: 77). Jefferys' aim was, therefore, somewhat distant from our own in re-analysing for references to family and community. Re-analysis, or secondary analysis as it is more commonly known, opens up possibilities for new theories, concepts, and data to be created from an original set of data. Our aim here is to outline Jeffery's study, discuss methodological issues arising from secondary analysis, and raise some ethical issues occasioned by returning to data, before identifying some new interpretations that specifically relate to family and community.

The Jefferys' data

Margot Jefferys chose a theoretical sample of the people whom she believed could tell her most about the development of geriatrics. As far as can be seen, she had a straightforward historical motivation to capture the experience of the 'pioneers' before they died. The oldest 'pioneer' was 92 in 1991, and 15 had been born before 1915. The theoretical model behind this approach appears to be that change results from the activities of key individuals. Though it seems unlikely that Margot Jefferys would have seen this theory as adequate for a full study, it is clearly embodied in the interviews and reflects the hierarchical nature of power in hospital medicine. The theoretical sample was mainly doctors (geriatricians, with a few psychogeriatricians and general practitioners), but the sample also included pioneering nurses, social workers, occupational therapists, civil servants, officials from voluntary organisations, and two ministers (Kenneth Robinson and Enoch Powell).

The interviews can be described as guided life histories. Interviewees were asked about family and early education in so far as it accounted for their going into medicine, but the main focus was their careers and their views on how geriatrics developed. During their careers geriatric medicine had moved from being a matter of rehabilitating bed-bound, chronically ill patients in former workhouses to visiting older people in their homes (to ensure they were being correctly admitted and that their relatives might be able to take them again after treatment), and finally to seeing relatives mainly in hospital with 'the community' now a recognised partner in care. These transitions were common to all interviewees' experiences, but they had taken place at different times. It appeared that all three stages could be found in Britain at any time up till the late 1970s. The interviewees describe their careers against the backdrop of changing organisational and recruitment practices before and after the establishment of the NHS. Many identify their own role in bringing about the relocation of beds and the movement of resources away from the old long-stay hospitals and towards models of care built on principles of rehabilitation and, increasingly, care in the community.

Secondary analysis

Writing as recently as 2000, Paul Thompson described attempts to identify methods for the secondary analysis of qualitative data as 'the silent space' (Thompson 2000: 3). Four years later, Thompson and Louise Corti pointed to the 'new culture of the secondary use of qualitative data' (Thompson and Corti 2004: 341). The intervening period had seen a rapid growth of interest in secondary analysis, with new projects, new methods, and new data emerging into what is now an established arena for debate.[1] Definitions were called for and Janet Heaton's definition has proved helpful, describing secondary analysis as 'a methodology for the study of non-naturalistic or artefactual data derived from previous studies, such as fieldnotes, observational records, and tapes and transcripts of interviews and focus groups' (Heaton 2004: 6).

There have, needless to say, been criticisms of the reuse of data. Principal amongst these have been those of Martin Hammersley and Natasha Mauthner and colleagues (Mauthner *et al*. 1998; Parry and Mauthner 2004). Briefly, the points these authors make are that data are 'constructed', the product of a particular moment in time and of a particular set of interactions which 'involve an informal and intuitive element'. More than this, the 'cultural habitus' of a researcher, their ideas, and acquired research experience makes it impossible for another researcher to understand their original meaning and interpretation (Hammersley 1997: 138–9). Hammersley also suggests that even when two researchers are very close in their understanding 'there will also be relevant data missing'; in any secondary analysis it is likely that this will come to be increasingly significant' (ibid.: 139). Finally, he argues that to go back with a different purpose undermines the importance of context, something that is particularly important for ethnographic studies because 'The fieldworker interprets [fieldnotes] against the background of all that he or she tacitly knows about the setting as a result of first-hand experience, a background that may not be available to those without that experience' (ibid.). Of course these arguments could apply to most historical documents which are also products of time and place, as are oral history interviews. Without opportunities for reinterpretation, much of what we recognise as historical research would come to an end.

Mauthner and her colleagues (1998) identify similar and additional problems. On returning to their own data, each of the authors finds that these were created in specific researcher–researched interactions. They also raise the question of missing data, pointing out that the original researcher, in this case themselves in an earlier life stage, did not necessarily ask all the questions that might have been asked. They also argue that their original research exists in 'the boundaries within which the fieldwork was accomplished (Mauthner *et al*. 1998: 742). This boundedness renders their original data unreachable. In presenting their old data as beyond subsequent interpretation on the basis of their historically embedded subjectivity, they criticise secondary analysis as 'naively realist' because it 'hoodwinks us into believing they are entities without concomitant relations' (ibid: 743).

Niamh Moore, in a robust response, challenges this rather protectionist attitude to old data. As she points out, the original data still exist but to rework them is to open up new possibilities for advancing knowledge in a different context:

> Their account, with its attention to the context and reflexivity involved in the production of the so-called 'pre-existing' data, proceeds at times as if

they understand reusing data to be about some attempt to repeat or reconstruct the original research project, as if it is another interview project, rather than as a new project in its own right, this time an archival or documentary project. They fail to appreciate the necessity of attention to the context and reflexivity of the *current* project, which effectively makes new data out of old. Ironically it is their mistaking of the temporality of the context and reflexive production of the data which underlies their belief in the limitations of reusing data. Their construction of the issues in this debate consistently leaves the data behind in the past, in the original project that produced the data.

(Moore 2006)

Creating new data from old offers intriguing possibilities which make practising secondary data analysis so attractive. In an earlier paper, one of us has already shown how a new reading of the Jefferys' data has led to new research questions and a new focus for that data. The pioneers of geriatric medicine were reliant on recruitment of doctors from South Asia to build up their departments. This was not a focus of the original set of interviews, but becomes obvious after a new reading of the data (Bornat 2003). Though Jefferys and her interviewees were focusing on the roles and careers of a particular medical elite, the contribution of more junior doctors, many of whom were overseas-trained and (initially, at least) occupied a more lowly status, was only mentioned in passing:

> ... staffing geriatric departments hasn't always been easy, we have had to appoint quite a lot of doctors from the Indian sub-continent to be registrars and even senior registrars, so for quite a period the only applicants for consultant jobs were in fact not British citizens trained by British methods. They had been to respectable geriatric departments and learnt the trade but when they got appointed to x, y, z, they had Indian or Pakistani names or whatever else. And it tended to get known as the sort of, you know, dark-skinned specialty.
> (John Agate, born 1919, British Library catalogue C512/8/01–02)

By addressing questions about ethnicity, new data emerged about the origins of the specialty and with it a different take on the role and influence of the pioneers. This is an area where the historical context has changed greatly over the last half-century. Awareness of discrimination, the uses and abuses of language, and the political and legal frameworks that support equal opportunities have developed in ways that impoverish interpretations of meaning that ignore the historical context (Bornat 2005 and Evans and Thane 2006 for discussions of changed language use and revisiting data).

However, the questions of 'missing data' and the contexts of their collection cannot be avoided. In our case, re-analysis of what was said about family and community was relatively unproblematic. Neither was the main focus of the original interviews, so what the geriatricians had to say about them was either in response to one question (see below) or spontaneous mentions initiated as part of their general view of their role in geriatric medicine.

Missing data may arise simply because questions were not asked at the time of the original data set, but that begs the question of how this came to happen. Oral historians, and others who may use biographical material, often puzzle over the issue of 'silence' in the data. It is most commonly addressed in relation to assumptions about suppression, often with the implication that this follows from deliberate or unconscious self-censorship. Luisa Passerini began the debate amongst oral historians in her study of working-class remembering of the Fascist period in Italy. She heard people making only passing references to Fascism, or who apparently had selective recall, neglecting the detail of their daily lives, without a hint of what it was like to live surrounded by Fascist organisations and institutions (Passerini 1979). Subsequently, discussions about silence have tended to focus more on the insights of the interviewer or interpreter to make sense of what is heard or read (Moodie 2000; Roper 2003; Parr 2007). However, Passerini's conclusion was rather different. She argues that silences and omissions should more accurately be attributed to 'incorrect formulations of problems' (Passerini 1979: 92). Secondary analysis offers the possibility of identifying what the missing questions might have been, or the limited nature of their formulation, and going further to ask new questions of the data, developing and extending the original focus of research.

In contrast to this important point made by Passerini, in the argument set out below, we are identifying a set of discourses on the concepts of family and community in geriatric medicine that were spontaneously produced by interviewees, even though the original data collectors did not ask for them. At this point in time we cannot know whether so few questions were asked because the interviewers shared an understanding of the place of family and community in geriatric medicine which was taken for granted, or because the researchers were genuinely uninterested in that aspect of the development of the speciality.

Ethical issues

Long semi-structured, typewritten interviews need a great deal of work if they are to be reused in social research. However, digitalisation produces a new body of data that can be searched digitally, opening up a vast range of new possibilities and ethical problems. The first ethical issue is one of consent. The participants in the Jefferys' study had agreed to cooperate with a highly respected retired medical sociologist who had participated in most of the developments they described. They were willing to place their lifetime's achievement on record in the British Library Sound Archive for all to access. The interviews were impeccably conducted. The researchers obtained oral and written consent, tapes were transcribed using a manual typewriter, and tapes and transcriptions were placed in the Sound Archive along with summaries of each interview. Informed consent had been given for a personal life history with emphasis on contributions to British geriatric medicine. At the time of interview additional data such as published papers, photos, and other documents were also collected if they were offered. Some participants, though we do not know whom or how many, also read through the transcripts of their interviews and corrected them before they went onto public display. Legally, therefore, there are no ethical issues involved in re-accessing and re-analysing these data.

However, the British Sociological Association's ethical guidelines state that:

> As far as possible participation in sociological research should be based on the freely given *informed* (our emphasis) consent of those studied. This implies a responsibility on the sociologist to explain in appropriate detail, and in terms meaningful to participants, what the research is about, who is undertaking and financing it, why it is being undertaken, and how it is to be disseminated and used.
>
> (British Sociological Association 2002)

This leaves open the question of future uses, funded by different bodies, with different research agendas. The guidelines go on to say that:

> Sociologists should be careful, on the one hand, not to give unrealistic guarantes of confidentiality and, on the other, not to permit communication of research films or *records* (our emphasis) to audiences other than those to which the research participants have agreed.
>
> (ibid.)

Still more problematic,

> Where there is a likelihood that data may be shared with other researchers, the potential uses to which the data might be put must be discussed with research participants and their consent obtained for the future use of the material.
>
> (ibid.)

The original researchers were very clearly focused on one purpose and it seems likely that, when agreeing to be part of the British Library Sound Archive, the respondents understood that their words might be analysed by a range of researchers concerned with different aspects of medical history or medical sociology. Some respondents were aware of the tape recorder and even deliberately spoke off record, but there is no evidence that they were thinking of others using their life stories for different purposes in the future. There is no record of discussion about the ways in which the values of future researchers, their areas of interest, the language used, and the interpretations thought viable would change over the coming decades. It was clear that informed consent did not, and could not, have included a full discussion of potential uses for the data.

However, we have to note that there are fundamental limits to informed consent and the circumstances in which it can realistically be obtained. For example, it is almost certainly impossible to obtain when face-to-face interviews cover highly personal or emotive subjects; neither the interviewer nor the respondent can be sure how an interview will develop in such circumstances. It is good practice to make it clear that outcomes of such an interview cannot be predicted, and in some cases even to point out that the researcher has an overriding ethical duty to report illegal activities. The respondent should at least be warned and know to avoid certain subjects – but this is no guarantee that they will not be mentioned, or that other painful and identity threatening issues will not be raised. Consent may be freely given and even maintained after such an interview – especially if the experience was felt to be therapeutic (Bornat 2001) – but it will not have been 'informed' consent prior to the interview. Both participants and interviewers may know they are at risk, but they cannot be sure what the risk is and hence cannot be fully informed. In face-to-face or real-time interviews this problem can be partly overcome by allowing respondents to withdraw from a research project, but that may not be possible in secondary analysis when participants have died or cannot be traced.

A second ethical issue is that the ethical guidelines for oral history or literary biography are very much more permissive. Character assassination by a biographer may be deplored by reviewers, but as long as the analysis remains within the law it will not usually be deemed unethical. Oral historians with a tradition of identification with their participants are unlikely to upset or denigrate their informants (Yow 2006). The Oral History Society's ethical guidelines are also firm on the issue of informed consent:

> Interviewing people serves very little purpose unless the interviews become available for use. It is unethical, and in many cases illegal, to use interviews without the *informed consent* of the interviewee, in which the nature of the use or uses is clear and explicit.
>
> (Ward, n.d.; Parry and Mauthner 2004)

However, the guidelines go on to suggest possible avoidance procedures (mainly use of documentation, including copyright assigning, which can, at least, protect against future legal action).

The oral history tradition places great stress on the nature of the interview, its enabling and empowering qualities, and its sensitivity and an implied intimacy. Preparation for the interview not only involves familiarising oneself with the context of a person's life, their occupation, community, generation, and the public chronology of their time, but it also means developing social and interpersonal skills, listening capabilities, and empathy (Ritchie 2003). The result can often be a personal relationship that lasts over some time, but most certainly the result is a sufficiently close relationship that leads to changed perspectives on both sides of the microphone.

The responsibilities of the interviewer in such circumstances are great. Attending to these, perhaps through the formality of the release form and talking people through matters of ownership and rights to edit and change what has been spoken, means that the relationship between the researcher and the data is very different from that expected in social science. Some oral historians argue the case for a continuing sense of partnership and shared endeavour (Frisch 1990). Under such conditions and if, for the best ethical reasons, oral historians sign up to the notion of 'shared authority', will this make the interview a more personal and therefore private relationship, less accessible to a secondary analyser?

For the reasons discussed above we would suggest that for all who reuse qualitative data, the ethical issue is not informed consent but a duty of care to the respondents, and possibly to their descendents. Consent, preferably written, but in some cases as part of the recording, is essential. The purpose of the research and its potential uses should always be explained. The key points here are that there should be no deceit and that researchers should 'in so far as is possible' ensure that the 'physical, social and psychological well-being of research participants is not adversely affected by the research' (British Sociological Association 2002). This means that data which have been freely given for one purpose should not knowingly be re-analysed in a different context or in ways that would be likely to upset or harm the original respondents. The conclusions drawn from re-analysis should not cause 'physical, social or psychological' (British Sociological Association 2002) pain to the original respondents in the same way that real-time oral history research would seek to avoid causing pain. And if there has been a lapse in time, we must also ask how surviving relatives would feel. The upsurge in family campaigns to clear the names of grandparents, and even great grandparents, who may have been wrongly convicted of crime or desertion indicates a growing popular concern with family history and the ethical issues that are involved (Kean 2004). It also raises questions about changing constructions of what is meant by family, both over time and within the life time of a family member.

Family and community

The Jefferys' interview transcripts were scanned and cleaned, and the resulting texts were put into a form suitable for computer-assisted qualitative data analysis (CAQDAS) and analysed using the N6 version of QSR NUD*IST. Searches for topics relating to family and community were aided by the original researchers who asked two standard questions. The first was whether the family had maintained its caring abilities over the career of the respondent. The second asked for views on the NHS and Community Care Act 1990, which aimed to move care of older people from institutions into the 'community' (Means and Smith 1998). In most cases the researchers succeeded in addressing these questions in some form or other, but these were elite interviews and the content varied depending on whether the participants took over the interview or allowed the interviewer to lead the discussion. However, once the typescripts were digitalised it became much easier to find a fuller range of references to family and community, and to analyse a wider range of comments than those attached to specific words or questions.

The use of CAQDAS raises the question of context of text segments. Digital searching or coding can lead to quotations from interviews that are divorced from their context and so distort the views expressed. The solution is to check on the context by displaying the word, sentence, or paragraph with its surrounding text and as much of the interview as is needed to clarify the meaning. Researcher judgement will still be necessary, but this is inherent in any qualitative analysis. Other researchers have pointed out the rewards of working with CAQDAS, suggesting that the process is enlightening and helpful to the development of more complex interpretations (Coffey *et al.* 1996). What is helpful and confirming is, as Thompson (2002) suggests, to make the process as transparent at possible. Digital searching and coding therefore enlarged our sample of views on family and community offered by the interviewees.

The distinction between family and community arises partly because of language change (see above). 'Community' was not a word much used in the earlier part of our period when it was largely covered by 'family' in so far as the concept arose, but it became increasingly popular in the 1980s with the policy of closing large long-stay mental hospitals. In the interviews it was associated with the results of the NHS and Community Care Act 1990 (even though this had not then fully come into force). Respondents were limited by class, culture, and historical context in their perceptions of family and community. They were uniformly middle class, and 48 out of the 53 doctors were men, while most of their patients were women. In the case of the earliest pioneers, their patients were not simply working class, but severely disadvantaged members of the working class. They were old and they had been admitted to a building that was either the old workhouse or something very like it. The Poor Law, and with it the official designation of workhouse, ended in 1929. However, hospitals for the chronically ill were frequently part of the old Poor Law system, and popular folklore has only recently stopped seeing them as places where people were sent to die. Hence the lives of their patients were alien to the well-brought-up doctors who were suddenly faced with a layer of society they had not met before. This account from Dr Nagley illustrates this sense of social distance:

> And the VD department [of the workhouse] was part of the dermatological section, of course. The other doctor was a lady, and she looked after the female VDs, and I looked after the male VDs. It may surprise you, but male VD is a lot more wholesome to deal with than female VDs. When Dr Peacock was on holiday I had to do the female VDs, and equally she did the males when I was away. And really, I was horrified, first of all, by the coarseness of the women, the young women there, and their lack of any sort of reticence about their problems down below. Oh dear, it put me off for a long time, having to do female VDs.
> (Lawrence Nagley, born 1911, British Library catalogue C512/58/01)[2]

Another, Samuel Vine, describes a formative incident in his first job as a registrar at Fulham hospital after an education at Cambridge and Guys Medical School, and war service in the Far East and consequent late demobilisation:

> And she so she said, 'Now I've got these prescription forms for you to sign' and do you know, I was just about to do it and I said, 'Wait a minute, sister, I have never in my life signed a prescription for a patient whom I have not seen and I'm not going to start this afternoon. I will see all these patients before I sign these prescriptions'. And the sister nearly fainted at that point because this was the first time any doctor had insisted on seeing the patients. Well, I was shocked, amazed, appalled, saddened and very upset at what I saw that afternoon. I could not believe that, within the campus of one hospital, two separate standards should exist for treatment based solely upon age, 65 for men and 60 for women.
> (Samuel Vine, born 1919, British Library catalogue C512/68/01–02)

Virtually no one who mentioned 'the family' felt that it had failed or was failing. So, for example, the questions like the following never got agreement:

> You hear a lot of complaints that the voluntary and the statutory organisations have to make good because the family no longer helps support its dependent members, particularly the very old. Do you feel that there is something in that?

The respondents were very aware of popular discourse, but most stated that their experience of families did not bear it out. For example:

It was fashionable for people who knew nothing about it to say, 'of course, young people don't look after their elderly relatives and parents like they used to'. Well, of course people have been saying that since the time of the Romans ... If you're honest, it's incredible how marvellous people are. That was my view in the end. Of course, you came across the odd family who wouldn't be interested in mum or dad but when, when you did come across somebody like that it made such an impression on you, being so different from everybody else that you remembered that the more.

(Ronald Dent, born 1906, British Library catalogue C512/63/01)

Another example is that of Eric Morton:

(I) Went into hundreds and hundreds of homes, and saw what everyone knows, or should know - incredibly squalid conditions in which they lived. Saw how wonderfully they coped. Saw how very few families neglect their old people, *despite what you read* ... I found in Nottingham that the rural districts and the real slums were the places where you found the kindest people. The middle-class housing estates were the worst. 'We've got to get rid of Granny. She's dirty.'

(Eric Morton, born 1919, British Library catalogue
C512/4/01–02, emphasis added)

A few took a scientific view and pointed out that the family had changed over time due to changed birth rates and survival rates or the migration of children. Many pointed out that families could be over stressed, but they all agreed that the majority of families were as caring as they had ever been:

I've heard of people who've required relatives to sign undertakings that they will take somebody back at the end of respite care, which is a very odd thing to do because it really approaches the whole situation in a very paranoid way, and I think I've never found that necessary. Whenever somebody's been admitted for respite and they have not been taken out, it's been because the carer has either died, which is hardly their fault, or become seriously ill. And, of course, many carers are pretty ancient and frail.

(Brice Pitt, born 1931, British Library catalogue C512/42/01–02)

So we might ask 'What did the family mean to the pioneers of geriatric medicine?' In the first instance the family was central to their concept of geriatric medicine. They consistently saw their work as being about more than just a disease. Geriatricians saw the patient as part of a family and community. To some extent they shared this approach with general practitioners but they had the added status of being hospital-based. They saw themselves as problem

solving because they combined the diagnostic challenge of multiple patholo-
gies in older patients with an awareness of social needs; this set them apart
from other hospital-based medical specialties. The earliest pioneers who were
sent for one reason or another to old workhouses relied heavily on families
for their success. By working hard, examining patients who had not been
examined for years, if ever, and by converting the nursing staff to rehabilitation, these pioneers were able to get their patients out of bed and make them
mobile. Despite, or because of, a lack of social workers and other support
staff outside nursing, they then called in the families of their long-stay patients
and suggested that they take their relatives home. Just as they did not question
how it came about that there were old, rundown institutions full of hundreds
of bed-bound elders, they did not question the existence of family for people
who had been in institutions for many years. This is a question that needs further investigation since, if we are to believe their accounts of success, the
pioneers were undoubtedly able to find families and get them to take back
very large numbers of older patients:

> The staff, who had now been impressed with the desolation of treating
> the chronic sick, now were beginning to see and to look at patients
> from a new viewpoint: Shall we show this case to Dr Cosin to see what
> he can do about it? And this came our way and, of course, a lot of these
> patients continued to improve so that relatives who now came in with
> flowers and grapes twice a week were beginning to give the impression
> that 'Perhaps we can look after mother at home'.
> (Lionel Cosin, born 1910, British Library catalogue C512/41/01)

> We also saw the relatives, of course, how capable they were: whether
> the daughter was off work, whether she needed help. So that we devel-
> oped a much broader – coming back to the original subject – a much
> broader concept of care.
> (Joseph Greenwood, born 1908, British Library catalogue
> C512/31/01)

> I saw the relatives and I saw the home conditions, how they lived and
> how they managed. So I had a very good picture.
> (Hugo Droller, born 1909, British Library catalogue C512/10/01)

Dr Droller was entirely normal in that he thought a short home visit could
tell him all he needed to know about a family. This was a very limited view of
family based on the old certainties that women would care and that the real
issue was whether there were women available and if the physical conditions
of their labour were tolerable. The families were partners in care, but this
partnership was not recognised by the professionals in these interviews. The
goodwill of families and the labour of women were simply assumed. The

narrow view of family as having a duty to care was challenged by only one interviewee among those born before 1919:

> We used to think in those days that it was nearly ... would it be 1940s, I suppose, that if a patient seemed well enough, or border-line well enough to be discharged, you were really not doing anybody a service to discharge them, because there was very little in the way of unemployment pay and the family would have to support him or her without any pay, so that really it wasn't doing anybody a favour, so it was really kinder, so we thought, to keep a person who was ready to be well and could do some work in a hospital, in the hospital.
> (David Kay, born 1919, British Library catalogue C512/45/01)

However, once the old workhouses had been emptied, the aim of geriatric medicine was to keep patients moving through the hospital. This meant much more home visiting so that hospital doctors could be sure that admissions were appropriate – both medically appropriate and in terms of the possibility of discharge later. The interviewees who were most involved in home visiting saw this as one of the key aspects of their specialty. It also involved turf wars with other doctors including general practitioners in the community and consultants (mainly in medicine and psychiatry) in the hospital:

> Well, I spoke to all the GPs in the area and said 'Would you mind if I saw your patient when you referred?' And they all wrote back except one, and I convinced him. And then it enabled us to see the home, suitability of a home, whether it was a flat or a tower building or a cellar, or what the facilities were, so that it helped in the idea of discharge: could the patient go back to that home?
> (Joseph Greenwood, born 1908, British Library catalogue
> C512/31/01)

> Well I would guess ... what were we doing? About five or six home visits a week each, throughout our time in Hull. And it wasn't for emergencies, it was for people that there was a genuine disagreement or diagnostic problem. And it was very good to see people at home and see their families and see the set-up there. I mean they are a lot of value to clinicians in seeing the real world outside the hospital.
> (Peter Horrocks, born 1938, British Library catalogue
> C512/48/01–02)

It appears from the interviews that the number of home visits fell as geriatric medicine became better established as a specialty and as new ideas of community care began to spread in the 1980s. Other doctors became able to identify potential geriatric patients and the specialty no longer feared wholesale dumping of long-stay bedblockers. Visiting hours were extended and family and relatives began to be seen in the hospital itself rather than at home. The word 'community' became more common as the interviews moved to later stages in respondents' careers, but no one spoke of community as warmly as they did of family; the pioneers born before 1919 barely mentioned the word until they were asked about the 1990 NHS and Community Care Act. As seen from the quotations above, they focused on the family. Pitt, using the word community retrospectively, explains one aspect of the problem:

> The other thing that I well remember from Springfield, and it really still sticks in the mind, was that even my very good mentor had this attitude, which was that a good registrar did not admit an old person, and a bad registrar did. So the whole attitude of the hospital to its community as far as the elderly were concerned was that it was like a castle with a moat and a drawbridge and a portcullis, and a good registrar would keep the drawbridge down and the portcullis down and would fend off the elderly because those few who managed to get in were bound to stay, they were bound to be dumped by their families. There was a thoroughly paranoid view of the community as far as the elderly were concerned: there was a great anxiety that the place would be flooded with demented, old people.
> (Brice Pitt, born 1931, British Library catalogue C512/42/01)

The improvement in community services was a great help to geriatricians. It became easier to see families and community services as partners in the care of older people. The later pioneers mentioned good relations with social services as well as improvements in occupational therapy and community nursing. 'Community' was also a heading that allowed the needs of relatives and carers to be increasingly recognised, even though this was often in the context of greater exploitation. (See, for example, Finch and Groves 1983, with their equation 'care in the community = care by the family = care by women'.) Evans and Sanford, among the younger pioneers, saw developments in the late 1980s and early 1990s as positive:

> And I think one of the ways things have improved recently is that we've gone very much more sensitive to the pressures put on families and, I mean in the 70s there was a policy in many districts, including the one I was working in then, that if a family was available, or, more specifically, if there was a daughter available – sons didn't count – if there was a daughter available then an old person was not eligible for home helps because it was assumed the daughter would do it. This was terribly misguided.
> (John Grimley Evans, born 1936, British Library catalogue C512/64/01–02)

In the community itself there's been a lot of initiatives in terms of recognising the need for things like carer support groups to help the carers of the elderly. And that's been a main interest of mine, the needs of carers.

(John Sanford, born 1948, British Library catalogue
C512/14/01–02)

Once the interviewees began to discuss more recent developments, problems with attitudes to the word 'community' became clear. The closure of long-stay geriatric wards and their replacement by private nursing homes was not welcomed by these geriatricians. In medical terms they had two fears: first, that patients in nursing homes would not be referred for specialist treatment; and second, that frail older people living in the community would be sent directly to nursing homes without a specialist assessment.

What's worried us perhaps in the last four or five years is the return to the situation that when an older person becomes ill or disabled and the family can't cope, rather than seeking a medical or medical social opinion from the specialist who is interested, and who can help, and who will do so in a positive way, older citizens are now conveniently put into rest homes or nursing homes, and I find this very sad indeed.

(Ivor Felstein, born 1933, British Library catalogue
C512/33/01)

Or more bitterly:

They talk so glibly about developing community resources as they close down this hospital and that hospital, and we see so much human misery as a result of the betrayal of those promises.

(Alwyn Lishman, born 1931, British Library catalogue
C512/39/01)

Oh lord, yes. It is disastrous, in my opinion. The only reason for putting old people into nursing homes is to kill them off ... There is quite a good case to be made out for doing that, but doing it by deception and deceit, which is what they are doing at the moment, I think is disgraceful.

(Richard Benians, born 1906, British Library catalogue
C512/55/01–02)

We conclude with the words of John Clifford Firth (qualified in 1941), which link professional and medical change to changes in family, community, and society:

... the actual care of the elderly people must bear some relation to the community circumstances at the time. In other words, whilst the attitude, the conditions for the community, change, so it must alter and change for the sick. So nothing's stationary in this life, change will occur. And I think this change goes on, the change at the moment trends to be towards community care, and I would have thought the possibilities of community care in principle fine, but it's a question of how much physical labour or people you can put in. I don't think you're going to be able to meet the demand, it's impossible.

(John Firth, born 1917, British Library catalogue C512/60/01–02)

Conclusion

There are ethical and practical problems in the reuse of qualitative data collected for different purposes by different researchers, who have different value systems and different research questions. Some have gone so far as to argue that reuse is impossible and cannot produce valid data. However, we have argued that with an awareness of the ethical issues involved, and with attention to the context of the original research and the context of the actual data being re-analysed, qualitative interviews can became a valuable research resource.

The re-analysis of this body of life history data collected in 1991 has allowed us to look at family and community through the eyes of one group of professionals. As pioneers of geriatric medicine, both family and community were important concepts for the interviewees. The original interviews asked whether family care of the old had declined and about recent developments in community care. We were able to find many other spontaneous references to these key topics. As a result we have argued that to some extent interviewees' professional identity and ability to develop geriatrics as a medical specialty in its own right depended on their recognition of family and community. In the early days the word 'community' was not used, and the term 'family' covered the relatives of their hospital patients. There were very few community health and social services, and the earliest pioneers relied almost wholly on families to take back the inmates of the old workhouses to free beds so that the new geriatric medicine could be developed and practised. They also differentiated themselves from other hospital-based specialties by their willingness to consider the patient in terms of pathology and as a member of a family. They saw geriatric medicine as complex and problem-solving, and the problems were those of family carers as well as of patients themselves.

However, just as the historical context meant that community was not part of the early pioneering vocabulary, so these professionals took a very reductionist view of the family: it was assumed to be caring, and the work of women was rarely mentioned separately. As the specialty developed, home visits were added to the distinctive identity of geriatric medicine. Again, an understanding of family and community were taken to be key features of geriatrics, and indeed were the aspects that attracted many pioneers into the specialty in the days when it was still deemed a dead-end career choice. As health and social services for older people in the community developed, geriatrics gained new partners and began to place more emphasis on the needs of family carers, including a recognition of the work of women. However, the data were originally collected in 1991 when policy aimed to shift from care by institutions to care by families, or 'the community' (Finch and Groves 1983). Interestingly, several participants ruefully, and somewhat anxiously, reflected on their own situation now that they had become old. The interviewees were well aware that community care meant more patients in nursing homes and more strain on families. For some these were clearly backward steps that threatened the work they had done in improving care of older people. Others were slightly less critical but none could feel entirely positive about the term 'community'. This contrasted with their generally very positive view of families who were seen as doing their best in direct contradiction to the rhetoric of family failure that was so widely represented in the contemporary media.

Notes

1 See special issues of *Forum Qualitative Sozialforschung/Forum: Qualitative Social Research*, 6(1) Art 31, January 2005; and *Methodological Issues Online*, vol 2(1), 2007, for example.
2 The Jefferys' interviews are identified by their individual British Library Sound Archive classification number.

References

Bornat, J. (2001) 'Reminiscence and oral history: parallel universes or shared endeavour?', *Ageing and Society*, 219–41.
Bornat, J. (2003) 'A second take: revisiting interviews with a different purpose', *Oral History*, 31(1), 47–53.
Bornat, J. (2004) 'Chance as narrative theme or pragmatic function?: geriatricians recall their careers', European Social Science History Conference, Berlin, 24–27 March.
Bornat, J. (2005) 'Recyling the evidence: Different approaches to the reanalysis of gerontological data', *Forum Qualitative Sozialforschung/Forum: Qualitative Social Research* [On-line Journal], 6(1), Art. 42. Available at: http://www.qualitative-research.net/fqs-texte/1–05/05–1-42-e.htm. [Accessed 27 April 2007]
British Sociological Association (2002) *Statement of ethical practice for the British Sociological Association*. Available at: http://www.britsoc.co.uk/equality/63.htm. [Accessed 27 April 2007]
Coffey, A., Holbrook, B. and Atkinson, P. (1996) 'Qualitative data analysis: Technologies and representation', *Sociological Research On-Line*, 1(1). Available at: http://www.socresonline.org.uk/1/1/4.html.

Evans, T. and Thane, P. (2006) 'Secondary analysis of Dennis Marsden *Mothers Alone*', *Methodological Innovations Online*, 1(2). Available at: http://sirius.soc.plymouth.ac.uk/~andyp/archive.php. [Accessed 27 April 2007]

Finch, J. and Groves, D. (eds) (1983), *A labour of love: women, work, and caring*, London and Boston: Routledge and Kegan Paul.

Frisch, M. (1990) *A shared authority: essays on the craft and meaning of oral and public history*, Albany: State University of New York Press.

Hammersley, M. (1997) 'Qualitative data archiving: some reflections on its prospects and problems', *Sociology*, 31(1), 131–42.

Heaton, J. (2004) *Reworking qualitative data*, London: Sage.

Jefferys, M. (2000) 'Recollections of the pioneers of the geriatric medicine specialty' in J. Bornat, R. Perks, P. Thompson and J. Walmsley (eds) *Oral history, health and welfare*, London: Routledge.

Kean, H. (2004) *London stories: Personal lives, public histories: creating personal and public histories of working-class London*, London: Rivers Oram Press.

Mauthner, N. S., Parry, O. and Backett-Milburn, K. (1998) 'The data are out there, or are they? Implications for archiving and revisiting qualitative data', *Sociology*, 32, 733–45.

Means, R. and Smith, R. (1998) *Community care policy and practice*, Basingstoke: Macmillan. Second edition.

Moodie, J. (2000) 'Preparing the waste spaces for future prosperity? New Zealand's pioneering myth and gendered memories of place', *Oral History*, 28(2), 54–64.

Moore, N. (2006) 'The contexts of context: broadening perspectives in the (re-use) of qualitative data', *Methodological Innovations Online*, 1(2). Available at: http://erdt.plymouth.ac.uk/mionline/public_html/viewarticle.php?id17&layout=html. [Accessed 12 December 2007]

Parr, A. (2007) 'Breaking the silence: traumatised war veterans and oral history', *Oral Hisory*, 35(2), 61–70.

Parry, O. and Mauthner, N. S. (2004) 'Whose data are they anyway? Practical, legal and ethical issues in archiving qualitative data', *Sociology*, 38(1), 139–52.

Passerini, L. (1979) 'Work ideology under fascism' *History Workshop*, 8, 84–92.

Ritchie, D.A. (2003) *Doing oral history: a practical guide*, New York: Oxford University Press. Second edition.

Roper, M. (2003) 'Analysing the analysed: transference and counter-transference in the oral history encounter', *Oral History*, 31(2), 20–32.

Thompson, P. (2000) 'Re-using qualitative research data: a personal account', *Forum Qualitative Sozialforshcung/Forum:Qualitative Social Research* [online journal], 1(3). Available at http://www.qualitative-research.net/fqs-texte/3–00/3 –00thompson-e.htm. [Accessed 26 April 2007]

Thompson, P. and Corti, L. (2004) 'Secondary analysis of archived data' in C. Seale, G. Giampietro, J.F. Gubrium and D. Silverman (eds) *Qualitative Research Practice*, London: Sage.

Thompson, R. (2002) 'Reporting the results of computer-assisted analysis of qualitative research data', *Forum Qualitative Sozialforschung/Forum: Qualitative Social Research* [online journal], 3(2). Available at: http://www.qualitative-research.net/fqs-texte/2–02/2–02thompson-e.htm. [Accessed 26 April 2007]

Ward, A. (n.d.) 'Is your oral history legal and ethical?' Available at: http://www.ohs.org.uk/ethics/index.php. [Accessed 27 April 2007]

Yow, V. (2006) '"Do I like them too much"? Effects of the oral history interview on the interviewer and vice versa', in R. Perks and A. Thomson (eds) *The oral history reader*, London: Routledge. Second edition.

Chapter 8

The family and social change revisited

Nickie Charles, Charlotte Aull Davies, and Chris Harris

Introduction

This chapter explores some of the conceptual and methodological issues arising from a re-study. At the beginning of the 1960s, Colin Rosser and Chris Harris undertook a research project which explored the family and social change. It investigated how the family had been affected by social change since the early years of the twentieth century, and its findings were published in 1965 (Rosser and Harris 1965). Our re-study, which began in 2001, investigated the nature of social change and how it had affected families in the four decades since 1960. We did this by replicating, as far as possible, the original study in order to be able to compare the findings of the two studies. In this chapter we explore some of the methodological issues raised by our re-study and the extent to which such a re-study can contribute to our understanding of social change – both empirically, in terms of changing family practices, and theoretically, in terms of how social change is conceptualised. In the process we reflect on how studies of family and community (in particular places at particular times – or in this case at two particular times) can illuminate general theories of social change.

The chapter is divided into three parts. The first part describes the study carried out by Rosser and Harris in 1960, henceforth the baseline study, and the re-study, carried out just over 40 years later. The second part compares some of the key findings of the two studies, focusing especially on what they reveal about continuity and change, and discusses some of the methodological problems we encountered. The third part explores the implications of our findings for general theories of social change and suggests a conceptualisation of social change which is informed by empirical data.

The baseline study

The baseline study was carried out in 1960 and was designed to explore whether Young and Willmott's findings from their Bethnal Green research (1957) were peculiar to a particular working-class area of London or whether they could be reproduced in an area which was culturally distinct and heterogeneous in class terms. Rosser and Harris therefore adapted Young and Willmott's methodology for use in South Wales, specifically Swansea. Like Young and Willmott, they focused on patterns of residence and frequency of contact between family members living in different households in order to uncover the extent to which the extended family existed in a culturally and socially distinct part of the UK. Young and Willmott had found that women and their married daughters living in different households shared domestic and childrearing tasks, and claimed to have discovered, within the largest conurbation in the world in the oldest industrial country in the world, the continued existence of the 'extended family'. They defined the extended family as involving daily contact between kin. Rosser and Harris modified this definition, arguing that it is not necessary for there to be daily, face-to-face contact for people to feel that they belong to an 'extended family' and participate 'in relationships to kin beyond the intimate circle of their elementary families' (Rosser and Harris 1965: 219).

Using this broader definition, they found that, despite their sons and daughters being geographically less close, older people in Swansea received support from their children and other kin. They found that 'the maintenance of relationships constituting the extended family depended ... on relationships between and through women' and that 'this was true of all our social classes' (ibid.: xvi). These findings were remarkably similar to those in Bethnal Green, only differing in so far as in Swansea parents and married children did not form a domestic group, and as a consequence domestic arrangements were not shared. There was a grouping wider than the elementary family of parents and children that had the composition of three generations associated with extended families, but this grouping was somewhere between a social network and a co-resident group proper. This, Rosser and Harris termed, following Litwak (1960a and b), the modified extended family. They suggested that increased geographical and social mobility, together with the 'quiet revolution in the position of women' (Rosser and Harris 1983: 115) reduced the ability of kinship groups to provide support for their members, and pointed to the emergence of a 'modified form of extended family, more widely dispersed, more loosely-knit in contact ... and with much lower levels of kinship solidarity and a greater internal heterogeneity than was formerly the case in the Bethnal Green pattern' (ibid.: xx). It was a family form that fitted a 'mobile society' which was geographically, occupationally, and culturally differentiated. Their findings therefore confirmed the continued existence of 'extended families' in urban settings, but also identified trends which, if they continued, would lead to further differentiation within kinship networks, a reduction in their size and density, and, because of what they termed the 'de-domestication' of women, a lessening of their ability to provide support to their members. These changes were conceptualised in terms of increasing differentiation (cultural,

residential, and occupational) within kinship networks which was undermining the group solidarity that had previously held them together.

The original study consisted of a 2,000-household survey administered
in what was then the County Borough of Swansea, supplemented by
ethnographic research. As we noted in an earlier paper, 'The survey
included the key Bethnal Green questions about frequency of contact with
and distance of residence from various categories of the respondent's kin'
(Davies and Charles 2002). The ethnographic element of the study consisted of semi-structured interviewing and participant observation in two
localities, one of which was culturally Welsh and the other middle-class
with a less clear cultural identity.

Conducting a re-study: methodological challenges

Between the time of the baseline study and the early years of the twenty-first
century there had been significant change, both in terms of the empirical context and in the ways in which families and social change were conceptualised.
We conclude our chapter with a discussion of how social change can be conceptualised. Here we draw attention to the conceptualisation of the family
that underpinned the baseline study and the changing empirical context.

Conceptualising the family

When the baseline study was carried out at the beginning of the 1960s, structural functionalism was the predominant theoretical framework within
sociology and social anthropology in Britain. Underpinning this approach was
a Durkheimian conceptualisation of the members of social groups being
bound together by shared values and shared occupational status; hence the
concern of the original study with increasing occupational and geographic differentiation within families. This differentiation meant that families might no
longer share values which served to hold them together. In addition, the family
was conceptualised as precisely 'the family'. It was seen in two ways. First
there was the structural-functionalist conception of the family form most func-
tionally adapted to industrial society consisting of a male head of household,
his dependent female partner, and their children. Second, and flowing from
this, the object of study in research exploring the family and social change was
co-resident groups comprising heterosexual couples, their children, and the
connections between such groups living in different households. Although the
original study took place in this theoretical context, it was concerned with
exploring the ways in which people living in different households were linked
together by ties of kinship. There were no assumptions about the composition
of these households as this was a matter for empirical investigation.

Theoretical developments since the 1960s, in particular the influence of
feminist theory within sociology and social anthropology, mean that there is

now an appreciation of the variety of living arrangements which people enter into and that, even in the absence of kinship ties, these may be defined by their members as families. Thus the hegemony of the male-breadwinner model of the family at a theoretical level no longer exists; conceptualisations of how people live in intimate relationships, in households, in kinship groups, and in networks more accurately reflect the variety of living arrangements that can be observed empirically. Of course the 1950s and early 1960s were the heyday of the male-breadwinner family, so it could be argued that structural-functionalist conceptualisations of the family were merely reflecting this empirical reality. In either case, the way families are conceptualised has changed significantly in the intervening period, something that is reflected in the use of the term 'families' rather than 'the family'.

Empirical context and social change

As well as theoretical change there had also been change in the empirical context between 1960 and 2002. Some of the things that had changed were the boundary of Swansea itself, the voting age, and the willingness of potential respondents to participate in what was, in the event, quite a lengthy and complicated questionnaire. Each of these changes posed methodological problems which had to be resolved. With respect to the boundary changes we decided to survey an area that was as near as possible identical to that of the 1960 County Borough. The 1960 County Borough is now part of the new unitary authority called the City and Council of Swansea. The area to be surveyed in 2002 was therefore identified as that comprising the areas of the 2001 wards of the City and County Borough which had been wards in the 1960 County Borough. The electoral registers of these wards provided the sampling frame for the 2002 survey.

We were also proposing to analyse census data in order to provide information about economic, demographic, and occupational change in Swansea between 1960 and 2002, and our decision to use the old boundaries meant that official statistics did not correspond to the area we were studying. This meant that we had to produce census data for the area which corresponded to the 1960 County Borough of Swansea. This problem was repeated with our ethnographic areas, two of which were not coterminous with easily identifiable census districts. In the event, census data for these areas were kindly provided for us by the Planning Department of Swansea City and County Council.

Between the two studies the voting age had changed from 21 to 18; the original study included those who were old enough to vote. We decided to adopt the same strategy but this means that the re-study includes younger respondents than did the original study. It was, however, people's unwillingness to participate in research which underlined the difficulties involved in replicating the original research.

Our original intention had been to undertake a 2,000-household survey as in the baseline study, but our achieved sample was only 1,000. This was due to the much lower response rate (43 per cent compared with 87 per cent), reflecting the changed social context and possibly greater concerns about intrusiveness and how research data will be used than was the case in 1960. It may also reflect the fact that in 1960 there were many more people at home with time to spend talking to an interviewer; this is illustrated by the difference in women's economic activity rates between the two studies: in 1960 the figure for Swansea was 29.4 per cent while in 2001 it was 52.9 per cent (Census 2001). We think that this may also help to explain what turned out to be the over representation of older age groups and under representation of younger age groups in our sample; older people who are no longer in paid employment have more time to spend talking to researchers.

How we did it

When planning the re-study we initially assumed that the completed questionnaires from the original study would be available to us; however, despite searching the university library's archives, they were nowhere to be found. Apart from some data which had been preserved by Harris, we were not, therefore, able to revisit the original 1960 data and had to use Rosser and Harris's published account of the study as the baseline for our own. We did, however, have a copy of the original questionnaire. In order to facilitate comparison between the 2002 and the 1960 survey results, we decided that we would replicate the original questionnaire as far as possible, taking into account the changed theoretical and empirical context in which the survey would be undertaken, but that we would expand the ethnographic element of the original study to include four contrasting parts of Swansea.

Due to the changed analytical context, particularly in relation to the difference made to our understandings of social class and family-households by a consideration of gender, we had to modify several of the questions in the original survey. There were some that it was no longer sensible to ask and there were others that we added in order to gather information about caring practices, unemployment, and kin connections between households resulting from divorce and remarriage. Alterations also resulted from the changed empirical context in which we were operating. This meant that our questionnaire, although retaining the basic questions about residence and contact which constituted the bulk of the original questionnaire, differed substantially from the original. It included questions on household composition, employment status, caring responsibilities, children, partnerships, residence, patterns of contact with kin, and membership of organisations. We therefore used a modified version of the original questionnaire which contained the key residence and contact questions of the original survey. We hoped to replicate the 2,000-household survey, drawing a random sample of 1 in 57 individuals from the electoral register.

We had less information on how the original ethnographic part of the research was carried out. We therefore decided to develop a semi-structured interview schedule which would enable us to flesh out the bare statistics produced by the survey, and to undertake participant observation in various settings in the localities where ethnographic interviews were to take place. The ethnographic interview topics included who counted as family, the importance of family, the nature of contact with family members, family occasions, social networks, the nature of support given and received, and questions of identity and family change. The social significance of friends and neighbours was also included in these interviews and attempts were made to ensure that interviews were conducted with people living in a variety of different household types and living arrangements. The qualitative data generated by the ethnographic studies was to supplement the survey data, allowing us to explore the meanings attached to the patterns of contact and exchange between kin identified in the survey. It would also provide in-depth information about social groups, such as minority ethnic groups, who were likely to constitute a small number of respondents in the survey due to their being a small proportion of the population of Swansea.

We conducted ethnographic studies of four localities, interviewing 122 women and 71 men aged between 18 and 92 years; 17 of these interviews were with minority ethnic interviewees. The interviews were tape-recorded and transcribed verbatim. Of the four areas one was middle class and affluent, equivalent to Sketty in the 1960 study, one was the culturally Welsh area included in the baseline study, one was an area with high levels of social deprivation, and one was an inner-city area with a relatively high minority ethnic population (all the minority ethnic interviewees lived in this fourth area). The samples in the four areas were constructed using a snowball technique with several different starting points such as churches, schools, community organisations, shops, and personal contacts. As with much other research on families, it was more difficult to find men than women who would agree to be interviewed; this is reflected in the fact that 63 per cent of our interviewees were women.

The survey was administered between May and September 2002 while the ethnographic interviews were carried out between May 2001 and October 2004.

Key findings

Changing households

In comparing the findings of the re-study with those of the baseline study we find both continuity and change. Perhaps one of the most striking changes is

the decrease in the proportion of people who are in co-residential, heterosexual partnerships. In 1960, 76.2 per cent of the survey population were married
and had children; by 2002 the proportion who were married had fallen to
53.8 per cent, with a further 5.5 per cent cohabiting (see Table 8.1). Similarly,
the proportion who had children had fallen from 83 per cent to 73.3 per cent.

There have also been significant changes in household composition. The
proportion of single-person households increased from 5 per cent to 19.9 per
cent while the classic extended family (consisting of three generations living
under the same roof) declined. In 1960, one in five households contained
three generations of the same family, but in 2002 this had fallen to one in
200. Almost the only sector of the population where three-generation households remain is amongst the minority ethnic population – particularly
amongst Bengalis, who are the largest minority ethnic group in the city. In
the Bengali group, three-generation, patrilocal family-households are common. This family structure contrasts with the two-generation neo- or
uxori-local family households of the majority ethnic population and also
with the female-centred kinship networks that are common in areas of high
socio-economic deprivation. These changes can be seen in Table 8.2.

At first glance this table, which uses the categories of the original study,
suggests a *reduction* in the variety of household composition between the
two surveys. The original intention of this table was to measure the inci-
dence of extended family households, and to differentiate between
households in which couples lived with the wife's parents and those in
which couples lived with the husband's parents, there being a tendency for
young couples to take up residence with the wife's parents in the early
years of their marriage because of the shortage of housing in 1960s
Swansea. These categories are now insignificant and, in that sense, there
has been a reduction in the variety of household composition. Indeed one
of the differences between 1960 and 2002 is that young couples no longer
need to share a house with one or other set of parents in the early years of
their living together (Chapter 2 this volume). However, the category
'Parent(s) and unmarried child(ren), with or without relatives, but not

Table 8.1 Marital status of 2002 survey respondents

	Number	Per cent
Married	534	53.7
Cohabiting	55	5.5
Single	195	19.6
Widowed	120	12.1
Divorced	75	7.5
Separated	15	1.5
Total	*994*	*100*

Table 8.2 Household composition (%)

	2002	1960
Person living on own	19.9	5.0
Married couples alone without children or other relatives	31.9	19.4
Widowed and/or unmarried siblings without other relatives	0.1	1.5
Parent(s) and unmarried child(ren), with or without other relatives, but not married children	43.2	49.2
Parent(s) and married son(s), with or without others, but not married daughter(s)	0.2	5.5
Parent(s) and married daughter(s), with or without others, but not married son(s)	0.3	14.8
Married couples with other relatives, other than own children	0.5	2.6
Other relatives living together, not any of above	0.5	1.1
Unrelated persons	3.4	1.1
Total	100.0	100.0

Note: For 2002 sample married and cohabiting couples are included in married category

married children' has become a catch-all category in so far as it includes single-parent households and households containing reconstituted families. We are able to disaggregate data for lone parents, but to do so makes no sense when comparing our findings with those of the baseline study as no data on single-parent households were analysed in 1960. Moreover, only 5.5 per cent of our sample is constituted by single-parent households and to separate them out for purposes of analysing residence and contact data means that the numbers in each cell, once analysis by class, ethnicity, or indeed anything else is undertaken, are so small as to become meaningless. We anticipated there being a greater variety of household types now than there were in 1960 and, indeed, the ethnographic data show that this is the case. However, their proportion in the sample as a whole is too small for us to be able to develop any meaningful quantitative analysis of differences in patterns of residence and contact with kin. Changes in patterns of divorce and remarriage were often commented on, particularly by our older interviewees. Many of them found it hard to understand the living arrangements of their adult children and were saddened by the instability of heterosexual partnerships. Indeed it is from our ethnographic interviews rather than the survey that we gain an insight into the complexity of the kin relationships of reconstituted families and the way that relationships between ex-in-laws are often maintained because of childcare needs and grandchildren.

The family, in the sense of the proportion of the population living as a heterosexual couple with children, has therefore declined between the two surveys. Families, however, remain of great importance to people and, as we shall see, adult children still tend to live close to their parents and see them almost as frequently as they did four decades ago. Indeed one of our major findings is that although the proportion of the population 'doing' family, in the sense of heterosexual partnering and parenting, has declined significantly, the way they do it, in the sense of patterns of contact and support between kin, has changed remarkably little between the two studies.

Patterns of residence and contact

If we look at where adult children live in relation to their parents and the frequency with which they see them, we find that the patterns of contact and residence that were found in 1960 have changed relatively little. Women and their daughters are still at the heart of kinship groupings and there is an exchange of domestic services which maintains high rates of face-to-face contact. Mothers and, to a lesser extent, fathers are often involved in caring for their grandchildren, and fathers often provide practical support for their adult children when they move into their own homes or when they need home improvements. Adult children are also involved in caring for their parents; indeed almost a quarter of our survey population was involved in caring for someone outside their own household, usually parents. Here we look in detail at our findings on patterns of residence and contact in order to assess how social change has affected family practices.

Residence

Our findings show that geographical mobility has increased between the two studies. This means that members of potential extended family groupings tend to live further away from each other than they did in 1960. There is, however, a gender difference with daughters being more likely to live close to their parents than sons and a greater proportion of sons having parents living outside Wales. Furthermore partnered respondents live closer to their parents than do those who are unpartnered and, for partnered respondents, the gender difference is smaller. This can be seen in Table 8.3.

Comparing the findings of both surveys, we find a decrease in proximity of parents to partnered respondents between 1960 and 2002, which is more marked for daughters than it is for sons. There is also a substantial increase in the proportion of respondents having parents living elsewhere. There has therefore been a widening of the geographical range of kin, increased geographical mobility, and increased migration into Swansea between the two surveys. The figures can be seen in Table 8.4.

Table 8.3 Proximity of parents to respondent (respondent as child)

Percentages of all and partnered respondents with parent living outside the dwelling

Parent Respondent	Father to son		Father to daughter		Mother to son		Mother to daughter	
	All	Partnered	All	Partnered	All	Partnered	All	Partnered
Same part of Swansea	28.5	33.5	31.5	31.5	26.5	29.5	33.0	31.0
Other part of Swansea	26.5	33.5	33.5	37.0	32	36.5	35.0	38.5
Total within Swansea	*55*	*67*	*65*	*68.5*	*58.5*	*66*	*68*	*69.5*
Region around Swansea	4.5	7.0	5.0	4.5	3.5	5.0	4.5	5.5
Another part of Wales	14.0	10.0	10.0	8.5	15.0	14.0	7.5	5.0
Another part of Britain	23.0	11.5	16.0	14.0	20.5	3.0	15.5	13.0
Outside Britain	3.5	4.5	4.0	3.5	2.0	2.0	4.5	5.0
Total outside Wales	*27*	*16*	*20*	*17.5*	*22.5*	*15*	*20*	*18*
Numbers	109	69	177	108	135	101	214	141

Table 8.4 Proximity of parents to partnered respondents (%) (2002 data reworked to make a direct comparison possible)

Parents' residence	1960 Married sons	2002 Married sons	1960 Married daughters	2002 Married daughters
Same locality	26	31.5	42	31
Other locality	45	36.5	38	41
In Swansea	*71*	*68*	*80*	*72*
Region around	9	4.5	5	5.5
Elsewhere	20	27.5	15	22.5
Numbers	383	112	408	150

Contact

Geographical proximity is, of course, related to frequency of face-to-face contact. A comparison of the frequency of this type of contact between the two studies for respondents and parents shows that it has fallen for every category, but that the falls are not significant except in the case of sons' contact with fathers. This can be seen in Table 8.5, which also shows that 24-hour contact has fallen, particularly for daughters.

This decline can be explained by the increased geographical dispersion of extended family members. If those with parents outside Swansea are excluded then weekly contact rates with parents rise to around 80 per cent for sons and 90 per cent for daughters.

Table 8.5 Frequency of contact between partnered respondents and parents (respondent as child) (%)

Last seen Respondents	Mothers				Fathers			
	Sons		Daughters		Sons		Daughters	
	1960	2002	1960	2002	1960	2002	1960	2002
24 hours	31	25.5	54	41	29	26	47	35.5
24 hours to week	40	42.5	27	38	41	38	30	38.5
Within week	71	68	81	79	70	64	77	74
Week to month	14	17	7	10	15	18.5	9	8.5
Month to year		13		5		13		7.5
	15		12		15		14	
Over a year		2		5		4.5		10
Numbers	345	101	348	139	237	69	254	107

Source of 1960 figures: Rosser and Harris 1965: 219, Table 6.3. The 1960 figures refer to all married respondents with parents alive. The 2002 figures refer to all married or cohabiting respondents with parents alive.

Note: The questions in the 1960 and 2002 surveys were slightly different so there is only one figure for contact with a frequency of over a month for 1960 while the 2002 survey made a further distinction between frequency of contact of a month to a year and over a year.

These comparisons show that, despite increased geographical mobility, the most frequent contact continues to be that between partnered daughters and their mothers, and that partnered daughters see their parents significantly more frequently than do partnered sons. This goes along with the other continuity between the two surveys which is that, once partnered, men tend to live closer to their partner's parents than to their own. The only category of kin where there has been a significant fall in geographical proximity and frequency of contact is between siblings. This has two consequences: first, it affects the internal structure of potential extended family groupings which can now be represented diagramatically as a star (with parents at the centre having contact with children but the children having reduced contact with each other), rather than as a net; and second, it weakens the kin connectedness of the society, especially that of the locality.

These findings confirm that the trends identified in the baseline study – increasing geographical mobility and decreasing density of kinship networks – have continued into the present. They also show that the gendering of kinship roles is still very much apparent despite women's increasing economic activity.

In the baseline study, proximity and contact tables are not available for those who do not have children; they constituted 17 per cent of the original survey sample compared with 26.7 per cent of the re-study sample, which is a significant increase. Our data show that those with children live closer to and see their parents more frequently than those without children, but we are unable to draw a comparison with 1960 patterns as the data are no longer available.

Normative expectations

These patterns of residence and contact are brought to life by our ethnographic data which also reveal the normative expectations underpinning them. One of our interviewees told us that he sees his daughter more often than he sees his son even though his son lives in Swansea and his daughter lives in England. He explains this with reference to the fact that his daughter has children, and he anticipates that this situation is likely to change as his son and partner are now 'trying for' a baby.

> We're waiting to hear now. I think if this happens then I would see a lot more of him then. [Why?] Well simply because they would be, with the baby you tend to want to go out for a break.
>
> (P039)

The interviewee compares this with his own experience:

> When my kids were young I'd see my mum a lot more then because it was somewhere to visit, somewhere to take them out. Summer, beach, walking, and then the winter then you'd visit and from that point of view, yes, that's what families are there for.
>
> (P039)

Another interviewee described the change in his relationship with his parents since having children:

> I think their attitudes to me and Gillian have changed since we've had the children ... I think it's probably brought us closer as a family then, since we've had children and they've been more included in our lives. Before we didn't need them an awful lot.
>
> (F048)

These accounts suggest that having children creates a 'need' for parental help which draws parents and adult children closer together. Half (50.4 per cent) of survey respondents without children are under 30 which means that many have not yet reached the stage of family formation if, indeed, they are going to at all. If proximity to and contact with parents varies with stage in the life course then it can be anticipated that when and if they become parents themselves, contact with their own parents is likely to increase. Increased geographical mobility, however, may militate against this, and it was our middle-class respondents who were more likely to live at a distance from their parents. For instance, 56.1 per cent of middle-class daughters had mothers living in Swansea compared with 87.1 per cent of working-class daughters. Generally, the parents of working-class respondents were more likely to be living in Swansea than the parents of middle-class respondents. Contact with parents shows a similar relation to class; these findings replicate those of the original study.

Living at a distance from parents meant that kin could not be relied on for help with childcare. One woman described her own and her partner's families as dysfunctional because of their inability to help her with her childcare needs when her children were small. She had moved to Swansea and had none of her own family around her but she expected some help with childcare from her partner's family. This was not forthcoming.

> It's not a very strong support network ... It's difficult because my mother-in-law has remarried and there were problems with the children of her new partner. So, I don't know what's happened there but it's sort of formed a barrier to her own children and the normal care that she would give to her own children. I mean ... when the children were younger it was only very occasionally that she would even consider, I can count on one hand the number of times she helped with them. And that was quite distressing because my own extended family were [abroad] ... So you had to pay people.
>
> (P019)

This reveals the expectation that a grandmother would be involved in caring for her grandchildren, especially when care was needed to enable the children's mother to go out to work. It also points to the fact that in the absence of this type of support, childcare has to be purchased. Those who lived a long way away from their parents were less likely to be able to rely on kin to provide childcare and were more likely to be middle class.

Occupational differentiation

The other important trend noted by Rosser and Harris was increasing occupational heterogeneity within extended families, specifically between fathers and sons. Since 1960 there has been considerable change in the industrial and occupational structure of Swansea, resulting in an increasingly differentiated occupational structure (Harris et al. 2004). This in itself makes comparison of occupational data from the two studies difficult. In addition, the influx of women into the labour market means that, while the original study assessed occupational heterogeneity on the basis of men's occupations alone, in the re-study we have taken into account women's occupations. These two factors have had significant methodological implications for our re-study and we have written elsewhere about how we resolved them (Harris et al. 2004). One of the difficulties relates to social class. In the baseline study class was derived from the Registrar General's Occupational Classification (RGOC) and, although the way occupations are classified has changed significantly since 1960, we decided to use the RGOC in order to retain comparability between the two studies. The other difficulty was that in the original study married women were assigned the occupational class of their husbands and, given the low economic activity rates of married women, this was relatively unproblematic. Given the significance of women's employment and the need to take gender into account in class schema, we could not simply ignore women's occupations in developing an occupational classification which would permit comparison between the two surveys. We resolved this problem by coding married or partnered women's occupations twice, once on the basis of their own occupations and once on the basis of their partner's. We then investigated the extent to which these two classifications, which we termed male-based and non-male-based, produced meaningful class gradients. We found that they both revealed class gradients as expected; we were therefore able to use the gender-sensitive classification for the 2002 data in order to compare findings from the two surveys.

Changes in the occupational structure, together with women's increased labour market participation, must necessarily generate greater occupational intergenerational heterogeneity within extended family networks whether or not occupational mobility between generations has also taken place. In order to measure this and to be able to compare our findings with those of the baseline study, we adapted the occupational classification used by Rosser and Harris. As this was based on the RGOC it involved a basic distinction between manual and non-manual occupations. In addition, class IIIa (other non-manual) was distinguished from classes I and II (professional and managerial) as well as classes IIIb, IV, and V (manual) (Rosser and Harris 1965: 96–7). Data from the original study show that 31 per cent of male respondents were in different occupational classes from their fathers. The corresponding figure for 2002 is 56 per cent, and for all respondents is 65 per cent (a comparison of women's and their fathers' occupations was not made in the original study). This increase should not be seen as an indication of massive social mobility because of the changes in the occupational structure which have taken place in the intervening period. Rather it is the change in the occupational structure which has increased the differentiation within Swansea's potential kin groupings as measured by fathers' and sons' occupations.

The chief change in the occupational structure relates to the greater economic activity levels of women; 69 per cent of our women respondents under retirement age were economically active compared with 78 per cent of men. As we have seen, 59.2 per cent of our respondents were partnered at the time of the survey and of them just over a third of our respondents formed couples where both partners were in employment; 58 per cent of this third had partners of different occupational statuses. This figure may be compared with the figure of 65 per cent for different statuses between respondents and living fathers in the 2002 sample, and the figure for all fathers and sons cited above for the 1960 sample of 31 per cent. A more detailed analysis shows that the differentiation within kinship groups noted by Rosser and Harris now extends to the heart of the elementary family and, in a significant proportion of couples where both partners are in paid employment (36 per cent), women's occupational status is higher than their partner's occupational status. Just under half of this 36 per cent were in the 'traditional' situation of heterosexual couples where women's jobs are of higher status than men's, that is, where the man is in a manual occupation (IIIM) and the woman in a clerical occupation (IIIN). There is also evidence of a generational trend towards an increasing likelihood of women's occupational status being higher than that of their partner's, and a decreasing likelihood of this difference being of the 'traditional' kind (see Charles and Harris 2007 for a more detailed analysis). These findings suggest that the trend towards increasing differentiation within extended family networks identified by Rosser and Harris has continued and is now to be found within the reproductive partnership at the heart of the elementary family as well as in the wider kinship network.

Understanding social change

Our findings show that the trends identified by Rosser and Harris in 1960 Swansea have continued between 1960 and 2002 and that kinship networks are more widely dispersed geographically and more internally differentiated occupationally (Charles and Harris 2007). Because of the fall in contact between siblings there has also been a weakening of the kin connectedness of the locality. Despite these changes, however, there are still high contact rates between parents and adult children, particularly between mothers and adult daughters who themselves have children.

Data from our ethnographic studies show close-knit networks of kin and friends are still very much in evidence in Swansea, especially in working-class neighbourhoods and amongst the minority ethnic population, and that there is a cultural association of close-knit kinship networks with both the 'traditional' working class and with being Welsh (Davies et al. 2006). As Elizabeth Bott (1957) observed long ago, close-knit networks flourish where there is geographical stability and, despite the increased geographical mobility between 1960s Swansea and the Swansea of today, levels of geographical stability remain high and people are still engaged in multiple roles. We suggest that this is associated with the fact that a relatively high proportion of Swansea's population is working class (even in the twenty-first century 50 per cent of our respondents classified themselves as working class) and that, even in our middle-class neighbourhood, kinship ties, though looser, still tend to be locally based.

These findings suggest that those who develop what have been termed data-free theories of social change would do well to take into account the empirical data generated by studies which are located in place. Such studies throw light on the way social processes affect daily life and can also throw light on grand theoretical claims about the nature of social change (Crow 2000). Thus claims about the decline of social capital (Putnam 2000) and the disembedding of families from local social relations are, we would suggest, premature (Charles and Davies 2005). The decline of social capital may be a feature of social life in the USA or other parts of Britain with higher levels of geographical mobility (Savage *et al.* 2005), but their application to the urban villages that make up Swansea is more problematic. Similarly, claims that families and individuals are disembedded and that 'traditional' communities (whatever that might mean) are disappearing would seem, at the very least, not to be universally applicable. Thus Giddens's claim that social relations are 'lifted out' of 'local contexts' and re-articulated 'across indefinite tracts of time and place' (Giddens 1991: 18) seem hardly to be relevant to family life in Swansea at the beginning of the twenty-first century. No more does his claim that place only has meaning in terms of 'distant influences drawn upon in the local arena' and that the 'local community' has disappeared (Giddens 1994: 101). Contra Giddens we would suggest that a society in which all social relations and institutions were 'lifted out' of their local contexts is inconceivable. Rather, different social institutions will vary according to the degree to which they need to be 'embedded' in matrices of social interaction to function effectively. Our evidence suggests that families in Swansea are very much embedded in the local context and that place has meaning precisely because of the local social relations (of which kinship networks are an important part) which constitute it. Indeed, perhaps it is precisely that family and kinship networks constitute the local context from which other social relations (economic, political, religious, etc.) are being lifted out.

How, then, are we to understand social change? Rosser and Harris related the occupational and cultural heterogeneity that they observed within kinship networks to increasing occupational and geographical mobility and the emergence of what they termed the 'mobile society'. We have argued that these trends have continued into the twenty-first century. What has occurred since 1960 may be conceptualised as an increasing differentiation of the social structure deriving from economic differentiation at the level of both occupations and industries – one of the most important aspects of which has been the enormous growth in employment opportunities for women, leading to higher rates of female labour market participation. At the same time, changes in the industrial structure have led to a decline in men's labour market participation. The population is still occupationally mobile, but the mobility is of a quite different kind from that experienced by the 1960 respondents. This is because it is not the result of educationally induced increased rates of mobility between positions in a relatively stable structure, but of the rapid differentiation of the structure itself. At the cultural level these changes have been paralleled by the *de-institutionalisation* of the expectations and practices constituting the family with the result that issues that were once decided by normative rules are now left to individuals to negotiate (Finch 1989).

The term de-institutionalisation does not, of course, refer to a type of society but rather to a process of change whereby components of a pre-existing social structure are transformed. It occurs not merely because an institution's 'charter' (to use Malinowski's useful term) loses its legitimacy, but because the range of social situations governed by the rules based on the charter become so various that the rules no longer apply. The decline of the normative structure is preceded by the decline in the utility of the rules predicated upon it. Progressive structural differentiation is therefore the precursor of de-institutionalisation; both entail an increase in the range of choices faced by individuals, so that, by virtue of the choices they make, people become increasingly *individuated*. Families are made up of people who are increasingly individuated and, as a result, family life is made up of the unscripted choices negotiated by family members between one another (Beck 1992). As a result, de-institutionalisation combined with the increasing internal differentiation of family groups means that families as well as people are now increasingly individuated.

This does not mean, however, that we are in a situation of anomic individualism, which is often how Beck's individualisation is interpreted, rather we are in a situation of moral individualism. This comes across from the qualitative data which show that, although there is a considerable variety of family forms, people are guided in their actions by a morality which is far from individualistic. They take into account how their actions will affect those they are close to and also what expectations there are about how those who are close to each other should behave (Williams 2004; Smart and Shipman 2004; Duncan and Irwin 2004).

Conclusion

In this chapter we have explored some of the methodological challenges of conducting a re-study and some of the difficulties of conceptualising and measuring social change by means of a re-study. We have argued that both the empirical and theoretical context of a re-study differ significantly from those of the baseline study, and we have explored some of the challenges arising from these differences. At the beginning of this chapter we noted that the theoretical approach of the baseline study was that of structural functionalism, and that the family was conceptualised as consisting of a heterosexual couple and their children. Durkheimian assumptions underpinned the formulation of the questions that were asked about patterns of residence and contact and the importance attributed to increased differentiation within kinship networks. In the re-study these trends are continuing and it could be argued that, by asking the same questions, we have implicitly adopted the conceptual framework of the baseline study. Indeed one of our most important findings is that the kin connectedness of the area has decreased between 1960 and 2002 as a result of increased differentiation within kinship networks. We have, however, gendered the questions asked and added new questions reflecting the changed empirical context; in this way we have adopted an approach which is informed by feminism and which recognises the variety of living arrangements which exist in contemporary society. The strength of this study, which replicates as far as possible the original research questions, is that direct comparisons can be made and the extent and nature of social change can be assessed. Thus the variety of living arrangements, while signalling change, coexists with a continuity in patterns of residence and contact between family members living in different households. This results in a more balanced assessment of the relationship between continuity and change and is an important corrective to claims that family life is in terminal decline, whether these claims take the form of political rhetoric or theoretical elaboration. In other words, a re-study can ensure that the extent of social change is not over emphasised and provides a corrective to grand theoretical claims that family and community are no longer significant features of contemporary social life.

References

Beck, U. (1992) *Risk Society*, Sage: London.

Bott, E. (1957) *Family and social network*, London: Tavistock Publications.

Census (2001) ONS, London: The Stationery Office.

Charles, N. and Davies, C. A. (2005) 'Studying the particular illuminating the general: community studies and community in Wales', *Sociological Review* 53(4): 672–90.

Charles, N. and Harris, C. (2007) 'Continuity and change in work-life balance choices', *British Journal of Sociology* 58(2): 277–95.

Crow, G. (2000) 'Developing sociological arguments through community studies', *Social Research Methodology* 3(3): 173–87.

Davies, C. A. and Charles, N. (2002) 'The piano in the parlour: Methodological issues in the conduct of a re-study' in *Sociological Research Online* 7(2), http://www.socresonline.org.uk/7/2/davies.html.

Davies C. A., Charles N. and Harris, C. C. (2006) 'Welsh identity and language in Swansea, 1960–2002', *Contemporary Wales* 18: 28–53.

Duncan, S. and Irwin, S. (2004) 'The social patterning of values and rationalities: Mothers' choices in combining caring and employment', *Social Policy and Society* 3(4): 391–9.

Finch, J. (1989) *Family obligations and social change*, Polity Press: Cambridge.

Giddens, A. (1991) *Modernity and self identity: Self and society in the late modern age*, Cambridge: Polity.

Giddens, A. (1994) 'Living in a post-traditional society' in Beck, U., Giddens, A. and Lash, S. (eds) *Reflexive modernization: Politics, tradition and aesthetics in the modern social order*, Cambridge: Polity.

Harris, C., Charles, N. and Davies, C. (2004) 'Some problems in the comparative use of "class" as a descriptive variable at two different points in time', http://www.swan.ac.uk/sssid/Research/R&H/Working%20Papers.htm.

Litwak, E. (1960a) 'Occupational mobility and extended family cohesion', *American Sociological Review* 25(1): 9–21.

Litwak, E. (1960b) 'Geographical mobility and extended family cohesion', *American Sociological Review* 25(3): 385–94.

Putnam, R. (2000) *Bowling alone: the collapse and revival of American community* New York: Simon and Schuster.

Rosser, C. and Harris, C. C. (1983) *The family and social change*, London: Routledge and Kegan Paul.

Savage, M., Bagnall, G. and Longhurst, B. (2005) *Globalization and belonging*, London: Sage.

Smart, C. and Shipman, B. (2004) 'Visions in monochrome: Families, marriage and the individualization thesis', *The British Journal of Sociology* 55(4): 491–509.

Williams, F. (2004) *Rethinking families*, London: Calouste Gulbenkian Foundation.

Young, M. and Willmott, P. (1957) *Family and kinship in East London*, London: Routledge and Kegan Paul.

Chapter 9

Capturing locality change

The family and community life of older people

Chris Phillipson

Introduction

A central concern of sociology as a discipline is understanding the nature of social change, as it affects both individuals and institutions. In this context, research on the family has been a prominent feature of sociological work – partly because of the importance of family relations for socialisation and support, and partly also because family change is viewed as a significant indicator of wider changes in values and beliefs. A common strand in contemporary thinking concerns what is presented as the increasingly fragmented nature of family ties. From its previous position as a haven of security, family life is more often viewed in dystopian terms; marriage, rather than for life, appears as an interlude to moving on to other relationships. High divorce rates, the popularity (or reality) of living alone (or going 'solo'), and the growth in cohabitation are taken as representative of the challenge to traditional social relationships.

By way of contrast, sociologists have challenged some of the more pessimistic forecasts about the future of family relations. What David Morgan (1996) defines as 'family practices' may be changing, but the reality is almost certainly more complex than one of abandonment of the family as an institution; bonds may be loosening from one angle, but creating more options from another (Riley and Riley 1993). More complex relationships (illustrated by the term 'reconstituted families') may suggest uncertainty from one perspective, but represent a widening of choice from other points of view (Duncombe *et al.* 2004).

How to study and measure the extent of family change has been a considerable challenge for sociology. The accuracy of views about changes in attitudes and behaviour over time are difficult to assess in practice. Social scientists have a number of different approaches that might be used, including longitudinal studies, population-based forecasting, surveys, and ethnographic research. All have their place in drawing together an assessment of how family practices and behaviours develop over different time periods. This chapter reviews another type of approach to understanding family change, one that uses previous research as a basis for assessing variations in attitudes and practices over time. The argument developed in this chapter is divided into three main sections: first, the broad approach of using what are referred to as 'baseline studies' is discussed; second, findings from a research project using this approach are summarised; third, advantages and disadvantages of this method are evaluated. This chapter concludes with a summary of the key themes.

Community change and older people

As already noted, concern about the extent of change affecting the family is commonplace. This is especially true as regards the position of older people, where family support has always been regarded as central to their morale and well-being. First, research has examined the social world of older people as dominated by families; second, as dominated by friends and neighbours; and as a distant third (to roughly paraphrase the formulation expressed in the late 1970s by Ethnal Shanas [1979]), as dominated by voluntary and bureaucratic organisations. In this context, any apparent 'weakening' of family ties might be especially significant for older people, given the importance of other family members in the provision of informal or unpaid care (Victor 2005). The importance of family bonds in old age was established (at least in the UK) through community-based research carried out in the late 1940s and 1950s, notably in: *The Social Medicine of Old Age* (Sheldon 1948); *The Family Life of Old People* (Townsend, 1957); *Family and Kinship in East London* (Young and Willmott 1957); and *Family and Class in a London Suburb* (Willmott and Young 1960). These studies were carried out during a period when concerns were being expressed about the growing numbers of elderly people in the population. A variety of reports focused on the problems associated with population ageing, specifically its impact on economic growth, and expenditure in areas such as pensions and health (Royal Commission on Population, 1949). Closely related to this concern was anxiety that the successful development of a welfare state might undermine the willingness of the community (and members of the family in particular) to provide care and support to older people.

The studies listed examined the thesis that, in the context of a developing welfare state, families were increasingly leaving older people to fend for themselves. Their findings, however, presented a different picture. Most of the studies demonstrated the continuing importance of kinship and family life in post-war Britain. Sheldon (1948), for example, describes Wolverhampton as a society in which the old are an essential part of family life. He questioned whether the phrase 'living alone' was, in fact, of any value, given the high degree of residential proximity of kin to elderly people. Townsend's (1957) study in Bethnal Green concluded that, despite the devastation suffered during the war, the community appeared to be remarkably successful in its provision of support to older people. Willmott and Young's (1960) research in Woodford set out to explore the extent to which geographical and social mobility may have loosened ties between generations. In fact, what the researchers referred to as the 'surprise' of their study was the degree of similarity between middle-class Woodford and working-class Bethnal Green. In terms of regular contact and geographical proximity, they were led to the conclusion that 'The old people of the suburb are ... as much in touch with children ... as those in the East End' (Willmott and Young 1960: 38).

These different studies became influential in shaping a view of the family as key to determining the quality of life in old age. Peter Townsend in Bethnal Green concluded that:

> ... if many of the processes and problems of aging are to be understood, old people must be studied as members of families (which usually means extended families of three generations); and if this is true, those concerned with health and social administration, must at every stage, treat older people as an inseparable part of the family group, which is more than just a residential unit.
>
> (Townsend 1957: 227)

The linkage between older people and the family unit itself reflected the trend in the 1940s and 1950s towards what Wilson (1977: 60) describes as the 'heavy emphasis on re-building family life'; this emerged as a major theme in social policy of the time. Initially at least, judged from the findings of Sheldon, Townsend, and others, this appeared consistent with the evidence that older people were not just in touch with kin (often on a daily basis), but that such ties were available to provide different forms of assistance. Against this, the longer-term trend appeared to suggest a drift away from family support to older people. The relevant factors included rising social mobility, greater affluence among younger generations, and increased female employment. The move from the environment of austerity which surrounded many of the communities studied in the 1940s and 1950s (Kynaston 2007) to the experience of affluence in the late 1950s and 1960s (Sandbrook 2005, 2006) came to be seen as disadvantageous to older people. This assessment was most clearly articulated in functionalist social theory, which was influential from the 1950s to the late 1960s (Goldthorpe 1987). But it also appeared in other theoretical accounts, notably modernisation theory as developed in the 1970s by Cowgill and Holmes (1972). Social change was viewed as creating problems for older people, especially as regards their apparent separation from an increasingly dominant 'nuclear family' (Parsons and Bales 1955).

The argument which emerges identifies a tradition of research providing an account of what it was like to grow old within a mixture of working- and middle-class communities some 50 years ago. The research gave particular emphasis to the importance of the family as a key relationship in old age, one which acquired increased significance for the individual over time. Interpreting research literature in this way, this chapter considers how the research was used to examine the extent of social change affecting the lives of older people.

Methodological issues

Trying to measure change over a period of forty or fifty years clearly raises significant issues and problems. In this case, the studies concerned had used different approaches and questions, and had been shaped by different agendas influencing why the studies had been carried out. Therefore, simply replicating the previous research was neither a viable option, nor was it desirable, for at least two other reasons: first, social science methods have moved on and different approaches are now available for exploring the research questions involved; second, repeating particular questions raises issues of comparability of response over different time periods. Despite these problems, it still seemed valuable to work from the broad findings of what we came to call our 'baseline studies', contrasting them with the situation which could be observed in the same communities some five decades later. In one sense, this was the first and easiest step; the studies identified are (or have been) highly influential and have been read by most sociologists learning their trade. The question as to *how* these communities have changed is of compelling interest raising, however, difficult issues from the standpoint of social investigation.

An early decision was to try and find a research question which would reflect the assumptions of the studies involved, giving us a basis for taking forward the research. The starting point was the very general question: how different is it to be an older person now in comparison with the 1950s? In making sense of this question the research drew upon Frankenberg's (1966) observation that in this period older people were surrounded by an 'environment of kin'. This phrase seemed to provide a useful basis for research questions which could be tested through data collection and field work. An initial decision had been made that data would be collected in three communities: Bethnal Green, Wolverhampton, and Woodford. These were the key areas from the original studies and they also provided a good balance between different types of urban location: inner city (Bethnal Green); metropolitan conurbation (Wolverhampton); and suburb (Woodford).

How the research would actually go about measuring the extent to which families were still important in the lives of older people was an unresolved issue. A couple of options were available: using questionnaires which raised themes similar to those covered in the original studies (i.e. questions about experiences of support and informal care); or combining fieldwork with some observational work at a community-level. On the other hand, our research objectives had a fairly precise requirement: we needed to know the full range of relationships which were important to older people, and the place of the immediate and extended family within this range. Moreover, a technique was required which would allow people the freedom of choice when identifying such ties, rather than forcing a limited range of options upon them. Collection of such information would allow the research to draw some tentative conclusions about the nature of social change over the time period involved. Another view which emerged was that we needed to take account of changes in thinking about the nature of communities. The original studies had assumed that the key relationships for older people were contained within close geographical boundaries; we assumed that many of these relationships were now likely to be rather more distant – transnational in some cases, rather than just within the UK.

Perspectives from social networks

Taking these points into account, the research turned to consider the value of using a social-network approach to the collection of data about the relationships of older people. The idea of the social network is well developed within the social sciences, initially through work in social anthropology in the early 1950s (Frankenberg 1966; Mitchell 1969). Subsequently, Bott's (1957) research on the impact of network structure on marital relations was important in spreading the approach's influence (Bulmer 1987; Crow and Allan 1994). The application of the network idea has been extensive, varying from locality-based studies (Fischer 1982; Wellman 1990) to research on the personal networks of parents and their children (Cochran et al. 1990), and studies of older adults (Wenger 1995; Antonucci and Akiyama 1987; Phillipson 2004).

The network approach had a number of advantages for our research. First, network perspectives (in theory at least) make no assumption about the nature of the ties in which people are involved; the extent to which these are dominated by kin or other types of relationships becomes the focus of attention. Second, social network perspectives offer a practical and flexible method for exploring community life, enabling researchers to work with dynamic notions of what 'community' means to people (Crow and Allan 1994). Third, the network approach can be used to examine issues related to personal change over time (Antonucci 1985; Kahn and Antonucci 1980) and within different social settings. Fourth, networks can be viewed as providing resources which may serve different functions at various points of the life course and, in terms of our concerns, may have an important part to play in supporting people in old age (Phillipson 2004).

Measures of social networks have typically been focused around three types of research questions: first, the *exchange question*, exploring people who might have performed a service of some kind for the individual

(McCallister and Fischer 1978; Wenger 1984); second, the *role relation question,* focusing on people who are related to the individual in some formalised or prescribed way (Cochran *et al.* 1990); and third, the *subjective question,* focusing on those who are nominated as 'close to' or on 'intimate terms' with the person concerned (Kahn and Fischer 1980).

In terms of our interests, all of the above suggest significant issues for exploring family ties in old age. However, bearing in mind the thrust of the original studies which were the basis for our research, we took the *subjective* dimension as the key measure for investigating the characteristics of networks in each of the areas. Rather than consider a variety of supportive relationships, the study examined those whom the older person defines as having a central place in their life (what may be termed their 'affective' network). The approach taken was to ask older people to make their own assessment about: first, who was most important in their lives: and second, the role such people play in the provision of support. The method adopted makes no *a priori* assumptions about the nature of the network in which people are involved. Traditional bonds and other relationships may be equally significant, serving different purposes for the individual. The technique used in the study, originally devised by Kahn and Antonucci (1980; Antonucci 1995), collects information about people who stand in different degrees of closeness to the individual. Data are collected by presenting the respondent with a diagram of three concentric circles. With the word 'you' written in the innermost circle, respondents are asked to also place in the innermost circle those persons who are 'so close and important' to them that they 'cannot imagine life without them'; those persons considered less close but still important are listed in the middle and outer circles. Respondents are subsequently asked about a variety of support functions that network members provide or receive.

Sampling

The research was carried out in two main phases. The first phase of the project consisted of a questionnaire survey of 627 older people in the three urban locations. This was based on the selection of a random sample of people of pensionable age who were drawn from the age–sex registers of General Practitioners in the three areas (following approval of the project by the respective District Research Ethics Committees). The size of the achieved samples in the original studies was 203 individuals in Bethnal Green, 210 in Woodford and Wanstead (older people only), and 477 in Wolverhampton. The Keele survey aimed for around 200 interviews in each area, achieving 195 in Bethnal Green, 227 in Wolverhampton, and 204 in Woodford. The second phase of data collection comprised a series of semi-structured tape-recorded interviews with 62 people over the age of 75 who had indicated at the survey phase that

they would be willing to further participate. The purpose of these interviews was to examine the issue of change from the standpoint of a
possibly more vulnerable group of older people. In addition, we also conducted interviews with members of the 'younger' generation whom the
older people nominated as being important in their networks. A total of
19 such interviews were achieved, a further 35 interviews with Punjabi
and Bangladeshi elders in Wolverhampton and Bethnal Green, and two
group interviews (one with a Bangladeshi carers' group in Bethnal Green
and one with the Asian interpreters and social workers with whom we
had worked in Wolverhampton).

Key findings

The main findings of the research have been discussed elsewhere (Phillipson
et al. 2001) and will be summarised here before consideration is given to
some of the methodological issues raised. A general finding from the study
was that kinship ties have maintained many of their traditional strengths,
despite numerous social and economic changes since the 1950s. Older people continue to be linked to family-based networks; with contributions from
older people, these provide various forms of support. An important continuity with earlier studies was that female partners and daughters were still
central to family practices in later life, providing emotional aid and services
of different kinds. The conclusion of the research was that the immediate
family offers an important protective role to older people; the family is reas-
suring in times of crisis, plays the role of confidant, and acts as the first port
of call if help is needed in the home.

The research did, however, stress the importance of the immediate family rather than the wider extended family. With some exceptions (e.g.
particular minority ethnic groups), we found the extended family playing a
fairly restricted role in the lives of our elderly respondents. The extended
family does come together for birthdays, weddings, or anniversaries of various kinds. But this should not be confused with more direct or active
kinship roles. These, from our research, are somewhat rare as kinship relationships revolve around the immediate family (and often just one or two
ties within it), rather than including a large number of relationships and
stretching vertically through different generations and horizontally across
different types of relationships.

The above finding highlights an important change since the baseline
research. At the time of these studies (notably in Wolverhampton and
Bethnal Green) older people defined their lives in the context of family
groups. In Bethnal Green, a majority (54 per cent) of older people shared a
dwelling with relatives. In Wolverhampton, in the late 1940s, just 10 per
cent of older people were living alone. Housing circumstances, and different
fertility patterns for this cohort, contributed to very different experiences in

old age. In contrast, a major finding from our study is that over the past 50 years we have moved from an old age experienced largely within the context of family groups (some ethnic minority groups have retained this form) to one that is shaped by what Wellman (1990) has termed 'personal communities' (the world of friends, neighbours, leisure-associates, and kin). Close kin are still available and significant in the lives and networks of older people. They are also a major force in providing different kinds of support. We asked older people 'who is important in your life?' and 'who provides you with support?'. For the majority of respondents, the answer to both questions revolved around kin.

But the way kinship is expressed now is different from the way it was expressed 50 years ago. First, elderly people living together as couples are more prominent now than was evident in the baseline studies. As Lynn Jamieson has argued, 'the historical shift from "the family" to "the good relationship" as the site of intimacy is the story of the growing emphasis on the couple relationship' (Jamieson 1998: 136). Older people (men especially) view their partner both as a confidant and a source of support in times of crisis, whether illness or financial hardship; this is an interesting contrast with the tension between husbands and wives described by Townsend (1957) in the *Family Life of Old People*. This reflects a more general point about changing relationships between generations: no longer living side-by-side in the same street or house, and with a less dominant 'mum' at the centre of the family, couples have moved to centre stage. This has also produced a significant change in the relationship between parents and children that is highlighted by the desire to live in 'independent' households and maintain 'intimacy at a distance' (Rosenmayr and Kockeis 1963).

Second, friends are also more prominent in older people's social networks. The significance of friendship has been a major theme in the work of researchers such as Jerrome (1992), Adams and Allan (1998), and Pahl (2000). Our research found that friends were the largest single group listed as intimate ties, and they may play a substantial role in providing emotional support. For the never-married, friends were listed as important sources of help (one in three would draw upon a friend for help with most areas of support). For those who were married, friends appeared to have a complementary role to partners and children. The role played by friends may be especially important in middle-class areas such as Woodford where relatives are geographically dispersed. This was a central finding in the earlier study, where local networks of friends (largely organised by women) were viewed as having functions somewhat similar to the extended family of the East End (Willmott and Young 1960). Our findings suggest that the cohort of people who moved from the East End to suburbs such as Woodford has maintained active links with friends in the immediate area. Such ties are important in sustaining leisure and social activities in retirement, although in many cases (also as the Willmott and Young study indicated) this represents a continuation of a pattern established much earlier in life.

Third, while some children may live nearby, older people still face the challenge of managing relations within more dispersed networks. In some respects this is aided by the growth of new forms of communication. In the early 1950s, only one fifth of *all* households had access to a telephone (Obelkevich and Catterall 1994: 145), with an even lower proportion in pensioner households. By the 1990s, telephone ownership had become virtually universal (although it should be noted that 13 per cent of respondents in Bethnal Green at the time of our research did not have use of a telephone, compared with 9 per cent in Wolverhampton, and 3 per cent in Woodford). More importantly, the telephone has come to symbolise the contact which can still be maintained with distant children and siblings. The research found that one in three of our respondents had last been in touch with someone in their network via the telephone (not face-to-face). Growth in the use of mobile phones and email has further served to accelerate trends towards electronic contact rather than face-to-face contact. These developments may create pressures for those lacking access to other forms of communication.

Reflections on the research

What are some of the issues raised by the research and, in particular, by the approach of revisiting past studies? Here, a mixture of advantages and disadvantages might be identified. Past studies are an important resource, especially where they have exercised the influence represented by our baseline studies. The technique of going back to these to illuminate social change is, while challenging, capable of yielding valuable results. Capturing how relationships have changed is an elusive goal that requires the deployment of a variety of techniques. Contrasting the present with the past through 'return visits' appears to be an approach worthy of further development as part of this work, but it is not without its problems. Identifying what is a genuine change, as opposed to a finding arising from alternative assumptions or different research methods, is an important issue. Our own study reported that friends were a more important part of social relationships than appeared to be the case in the baseline studies. Different explanations might account for this finding. On the one hand, friendship might indeed be more important now than in the 1950s, especially among working-class respondents. On the other hand, were investigators in the original studies (excluding Woodford) really 'looking for' or concerned with 'friendship'? The focus of these studies was largely on kinship and the family, and other kinds of relationships were a marginal concern. So whether friendship really is more important is perhaps less clear than it first seems.

Second, social changes over the past 50 years raise issues about the validity of comparisons across time. This point can be argued both ways. Bethnal Green, for example, is a dramatically altered community from that studied by Young and Willmott (as another 'return visit' by Dench *et al.* 2006 clearly demonstrates). Around one in two of the population is now drawn from minority ethnic groups, of which the Bangladeshi population is of primary importance (Phillipson and Ahmed 2004). Such changes have been highly significant for Bethnal Green. Historically, the population was more homogenous compared to other London boroughs (Husband 1982). Given the nature of community change, it is legitimate to ask questions about what is being re-studied. From this perspective, rather than take 'locality' or 'community' as the starting point, an alternative would have been to consider particular population groups (defined by class, age, gender, and ethnicity) and focus on key transformations over the relevant time period.

On the other hand, studying the shift from a relatively ordered working-class community to one experiencing a considerable degree of fragmentation and division raises issues worthy of further investigation. Research in the 1950s provided accounts of a locality poised on the brink of major change. The first change was the Second World War, the reforms which followed bringing, as Butler and Rustin (2006) note, rising living standards and a measure of economic security. Yet to come, however, were the effects of three overlapping developments: geographical mobility on the family networks of those who stayed in Bethnal Green; in-migration from new ethnic groups (bringing significant changes to the social and cultural landscape of the locality); and the broader issue of what came to be termed the de-industrialisation of the East End (particularly the closure of the docks and port-related industries). Studying the position of older people in the midst of these developments provides a rich set of possibilities for social investigation.

Third, for this particular study, re-studying three communities (rather than one in greater depth) may have been overly ambitious. Each community had been the subject of major changes over the 50 years, and needed greater investigation than was possible within the resources and time available. In particular, a focus on one community would have allowed different types of data collection to be pursued: participant observation in community organisations would have been valuable; archival work could have been pursued in greater depth (though the research did make considerable use of local libraries who were keen to help in the work); and living in the community for a time (along the lines of the investigators in the original Institute of Community Studies) would also have been useful. On the other hand, having three contrasting urban settings was interesting in respect of comparing the position of older people, and allowed comparisons to be drawn in respect of the impact of these different environments. It is also the case that further studies were pursued as a result of contacts gained in the areas. A follow-up study in Tower Hamlets (including Bethnal Green) studied the family life of

Bangladeshi women providing intergenerational care for children and (mainly) elderly husbands (Phillipson et al. 2001; Phillipson and Ahmed 2004). The work in Bethnal Green also provided the basis for subsequent research focusing on the social exclusion of older people, working in urban communities in London, Manchester, and Liverpool (Scharf et al. 2002).

Conclusion

This chapter has reviewed the development of a research project that returned to three communities which were the subject of major social investigations in the 1940s and 1950s. Overall, the findings confirm that the family has retained its influential role in relation to the lives of older people. It is, though, a different type of family compared with that of the 1950s. Indeed, an important conclusion from this research is that talking about *the* family life of older people has become a more complex task. There are many more different 'types' of older people than was the case immediately after the Second World War, and many more different types of families (partly because Britain is a multicultural society). But the family in some form is still central to support in later life, even if this is often focused around a small number of family members. And other relationships certainly do matter, especially for those without children, those who are single, and those who are estranged from their family (a group about whom relatively little is known). And community also seems to matter. Community matters not because locality produces some kinds of relations rather than others; rather, we can use ideas about locality and community to illustrate the important social and economic differences that exist among older people and which change over time.

Overall, the message from the research is that family relationships continue to be a major part of growing old, but there are constraints as well (some of which operate through choices and others through the pressures of particular life histories and particular environments). Demographic changes will almost certainly lead, as Bengston (2001) suggests, to the increased salience of multigenerational ties. Bonds of friendship complement these ties, but also, in some cases, replace kin-based support. However, it is also the case that a broad range of social ties will be needed to cope with the pressures and conflicts affecting family relationships. Global changes associated with migration and increased mobility represent one major element.

Of additional importance is the tension between work relations and family support. Sennett (1999), for example, has argued that the new flexibility and mobility associated with paid work may have a corrosive effect on long-term ties to friends and family. His analysis suggests that family relationships may be compromised by the insecurities and anxieties affecting people in employment. This raises the important question of the extent to which the social environment appropriate for an aging society may conflict with the economic goals associated with advanced capitalism. Family groups and personal communities, as argued in this chapter, are traditionally associated with high levels of support to older people. However, this may be disrupted through work ties that encourage short-term forms of association rather than the long-term connections characteristic of family ties. This last comment suggests the possibility of new forms of social division and inequality in later life. Studying these through re-examining past studies should be considered an important element among a range of methodological options.

Note

The work on which this chapter is based was supported by a grant from the Economic and Social Research Council, reference number L315253021. A full discussion about the research methodology, along with the research findings, is contained in Phillipson *et al.* (2001). I am grateful to Ros Edwards for her comments on an early draft of this paper.

References

Adams, R. and Allan, G. (1998) *Placing Friendship in Context*, Cambridge: Cambridge University Press.
Antonucci, T. (1985) 'Personal Characteristics, Social Support, and Social Behaviour', in R. Binstock and E. Shanas (eds), *Handbook of Ageing and the Social Sciences*, New York: Greenwood Press.
Antonucci, T. (1995) 'Convoys of social relations: family and friendships within a life span context', in Blieszner, R. and Bedford, V. H. (eds) *Handbook of Ageing and the Family*, New York: Greenwood Press.
Antonucci, T. and Akiyama, H. (1987) 'Social Networks in Adult Life: A Preliminary Examination of the Convoy Model', *Journal of Gerontology*, 4: 519–27.
Bengston, V. (2001) Beyond the Nuclear Family: The Increasing Importance of Multigenerational Bonds, *Journal of Marriage and the Family*, 63: 1–16.
Bott, E. (1957) *Family and Social Network*, London: Tavistock.
Bulmer, M. (1987) *The Social Basis of Community Care*, London: Allen and Unwin.
Butler, T. and Rustin, M. (1996) *Rising in the East: The Regeneration of East London*, London: Lawrence and Wishart.
Cochran, M., Larner, M., Riley, D. and Gunnarsson, L. (1990) *Extending Families*, Cambridge: Cambridge University Press.
Cowgill, D. and Holmes, D. (eds) (1972) *Ageing and Modernisation*, New York: Appleton-Century-Crofts.
Crow, G. and Allan, G. (1994) *Community Life: An Introduction to Local Social Relations*, Hemel Hempstead: Harvester Wheatsheaf.
Dench, G., Gavron, K. and Young, M. (2006) *The New East End: Kinship, Race and Conflict*, London: Profile Books.

Duncombe, J., Harrison, K., Allan, G. and Marsden, D. (2004) *The State of Affairs*, New York: Lawrence Erlbaum.

Fischer, C. S. (1982) *To Dwell Amongst Friends*, Chicago: University of Chicago Press.

Frankenberg, R. (1966) *Communities in Britain*, Harmondsworth: Penguin Books.

Goldthorpe, J. E. (1987) *Family Life in Western Societies*, Cambridge: Cambridge University Press.

Husband, C. (1982) 'East End Racism 1900–1980', *London Journal*, 8: 3–26.

Jamieson, L. (1998) *Intimacy: Personal Relationships in Modern Societies*, Cambridge: Polity Press.

Jerrome, D. (1992) *Good Company: an Anthropological Study of Older People in Groups*, Edinburgh: Edinburgh University Press.

Kahn, R. and Antonucci, T. (1980) 'Convoys over the Life Course: Attachment, Roles and Social Support', in P. B. Baltes and O. Brim (eds), *Life-Span Development and Behaviour*, vol. 3, New York: Academic Press.

Kynaston, D. (2007) *Austerity Britain 1945–1951*, London: Bloomsbury.

McCallister, L. and Fischer, C. (1978) 'A Procedure for Surveying Personal Networks', *Sociological Methods and Research*, 7: 131–47.

Mitchell, J. C. (ed.) (1969) *Social Networks in Urban Communities*, Manchester: Manchester University Press.

Morgan, D. (1996) *Family Practices*, Oxford: Polity Press.

Obelkevich, J. and Catterall, P. (1994) *Understanding Post-war British Society*, London: Routledge.

Pahl, R. (2000) *On Friendship*, Oxford: Polity Press.

Parsons, T. and Bales, R. F. (1955) *Family, Socialisation and Interaction Processes*, London: Routledge and Kegan Paul.

Phillipson, C. (2004) 'Social Networks and Social Support in Later Life', in Allan, G. and Morgan, D. (eds) *Social Networks and Social Exclusion: Sociological and Policy Perspectives*, Aldershot: Ashgate.

Phillipson, C. and Ahmed, N. (2004) 'Transnational Communities, Migration and Changing Identities in Later Life: A New Research Agenda', in Daatland, S. O. and Biggs, S. (eds). *Ageing and Diversity*, Bristol: Policy Press.

Phillipson, C. Bernard, M., Phillips, J. and Ogg, J. (2001) *The Family and Community Life of Older People*, London: Routledge.

Riley, M. W. and Riley, J. W. jr (1993) 'Connections: Kin and Cohort', in Bengston, V. L. and Achenbaum, W. A. (eds) *The Changing Contract Across Generations*, New York: Aldine De Gruyter.

Rosenmayr, L. and Kockeis, E. (1963) 'Propositions for a Sociological Theory of Ageing and the Family', *International Social Science Journal*, 15: 410–26.

Royal Commission on Population (1949) Report, London: HMSO.

Sandbrook, D. (2005) *Never Had It So Good: A History of Britain from Suez to the Beatles*, London: Little, Brown.

Sandbrook, D. (2006) *White Heat: A History of Britain in the Swinging Sixties*, London: Little, Brown.

Scharf T., Phillipson C., Smith A. E. and Kingston P. (2002) *Growing Older in Socially Deprived Areas: Social Exclusion in Later Life*, London: Help the Aged.

Sennett, R. (1999) *The Corrosion of Character*, London: W. W. Norton and Company.

Shanas, E. (1979) 'The Family as a Social Support System in Old Age', *The Gerontologist*, 19(2): 169–74.

Sheldon, J. H. (1948) *The Social Medicine of Old Age*, Oxford: Oxford University Press.

Townsend, P. (1957) *The Family Life of Old People*, London: Routledge.

Victor, C. (2005) *The Social Context of Ageing*, London: Routledge.

Wellman, B. (1990) 'The Place of Kinfolk in Personal Community Settings', in B. Wellman (ed.) *Families in Community Settings: Interdisciplinary Settings*, New York: Haworth Press.

Wenger, G. C. (1984) *The Supportive Network*, London: George Allen and Unwin.

Wenger, G. C. (1995) 'A Comparison of Urban with Rural Networks in North Wales', *Ageing and Society*, 15: 59–82.

Willmott, P. and Young, M. (1960) *Family and Class in a London Suburb*, London: Routledge and Kegan Paul.

Wilson, E. (1977) *Women and the Welfare State*, London: Tavistock Books.

Young, M. and Willmott, P. (1957) *Family and Kinship in East London*, London: Routledge and Kegan Paul.

Chapter 10

The UK Millennium Cohort Study

The circumstances of early motherhood

Denise Hawkes[1]

Introduction

This chapter provides a description of the Millennium Cohort Study, its design, and its history, showing how birth cohort studies can be used as a methodology to understand family, community, and social change. It also presents some results using data from the first two sweeps of the Millennium Cohort Study considering the family background and circumstances of the children's mothers and their relationship to the age at which they had their first birth of child in order to provide an example of the substance of change.

What is a cohort study? How can it be used to understand family, community, and social change?

A cohort study is a form of longitudinal study constructed by taking repeated observations from the same sample over time. A birth cohort identifies individuals at birth and follows these individuals through time, periodically collecting information on these same individuals. Birth cohort studies therefore build up a wealth of information which can be used to consider individual, family, community, and social change. (For a complete discussion of the birth cohort designs see Bynner 2004.)

The benefit of a cohort study over a cross-sectional study is that individual, family, community, and social change can be considered in response to changes over the life course. Cross-sectional data may be largely limited to describing population phenomena as the sample has data collected from it at only one point in time and cannot reveal changes through time of the same individuals. However, longitudinal data, collected at multiple points in time, can do this as well as describing a snapshot of the population so it can be used to elucidate the causes of phenomena and processes behind them. Longitudinal data allows information on events earlier in the life course to be used to explain current events. The sequencing of these events can help to dispel uncertainty about the direction of causality which is present in cross-sectional data. With longitudinal data, changes over the life course can be considered in terms of observations in previous sweeps, the current sweep, and changes between the sweeps.

It has been shown elsewhere that children in the Millennium Cohort whose mothers had entered parenthood at a young age found themselves in disadvantaged circumstances (Hawkes *et al.* 2004). This chapter considers the association between a child's mother's age at first birth and circumstances which preceded it. As the Millennium Cohort Study develops, with successive sweeps of data, the life course of the child can be considered from this starting point.

What are the Millennium Cohort Study and the other UK cohort studies? How can they be used to understanding family, community, and social change?

The Millennium Cohort Study is the fourth of Britain's family of birth cohort studies. Each of the four cohort studies has taken a sample of people born right across the whole country in a year and follows them from birth until, in principle, death or emigration. This well-established collection of national longitudinal studies cannot be found in any other country in the world. The cohort studies started with the MRC National Survey of Health and Development (NSHD), which is housed at University College London. It initially considered 16,500 children born in one week in 1946 in Great Britain. The NSHD then followed up a representative sample of 5,362 cohort members who have been studied 21 times to date. (Further details of the NSHD sample can be found in Wadsworth 1991.)

The second is the National Child Development Study (NCDS), which is housed at the Centre for Longitudinal Studies, Institute of Education, University of London. It initially considered almost 17,500 babies born in one week in 1958 in Great Britain in the Perinatal Mortality Survey (PMS). The NCDS has followed up this sample and they have been studied eight times to date. (See Shepherd 1995; Plewis *et al.* 2004a; Hawkes and Plewis 2006 for more information about the NCDS.)

The third is the 1970 British Cohort Study (BCS70), which is also housed at the Centre for Longitudinal Studies. It initially considered nearly 17,200 babies born in one week in 1970 in the United Kingdom in the British Birth Survey (BBS). The BCS70 followed up those in Great Britain (England, Wales, and Scotland) six times to date. (See Plewis *et al.* 2004a for more information about the BCS70.)

The fourth is the Millennium Cohort Study (MCS), which is also housed at the Centre for Longitudinal Studies. It drew a sample of 18,818 children born in the UK between September 2000 and January 2002. The initial survey was undertaken when the children were nine months old.

Two follow-up surveys have been undertaken: when the children were three and five years old. An additional follow-up is planned for when the children are seven years old. (See Hansen 2006; Plewis *et al.* 2004b for more information about the MCS.)

The Millennium Cohort Study is designed to be comparable to the previous studies and to make it possible to consider the impact of a change in individual, family, or social factors on individual outcomes. This can be achieved in two ways. First, the researcher will be able to consider individual or family change using the Millennium Cohort sample alone and look at those who over their life course experience individual, family, community, or social change. For example, a researcher can consider the impact of a change which affects the size of the family in which they live (e.g. the loss of a parent or the addition of a new sibling) on the outcomes for the cohort member and their family.

Second, the researcher can consider community or social change by comparing the different cohorts at the same age. For example, by looking at the BCS70 participants at age five and the MCS cohort members at age five the researcher can consider the effect of living in social housing on educational achievement. Note that we would expect to find differences in the types of children and families found in social housing across the two cohorts as those who experience social housing today are possibly a more homogeneous and socially disadvantaged group than those who experienced social housing in the 1970s. This social change could be because of the 'right to buy' policy introduced by the Housing Act which came into force in October 1980. (See Ferri *et al.* 2003 for examples of these types of cross-cohort comparisons for the first three cohort studies of NSHD, NCDS, and BCS70.)

Each of these four cohort studies are large quantitative studies. While this enables the researcher to attempt to describe a population phenomenon and elucidate causes of the phenomenon observed, the understanding of the actions observed are left to qualitative studies. Some qualitative and additional sub-studies surveys have been undertaken to supplement the main follow-up surveys in all the national cohort studies. For example, additional contextual information on the local area was collected in the MCS Health Visitors Survey (Brassett-Grundy *et al.* 2004). The use of qualitative studies in understanding family, community, and social change are described elsewhere (Chapters 7, 8, and 9 this volume).

How is the Millennium Cohort Study different from its predecessors?

The Millennium Cohort Study is different in design from the previous cohort studies in several important ways. These differences throw light on individual, family, community, and social change in additional dimensions which are not possible in the previous cohort studies.

First, it is the first national cohort study designed to ensure sufficient samples of ethnic minority participants, those from disadvantaged backgrounds, and those living in the Celtic countries of the UK, including Northern Ireland. Such participants have not been included in previous follow-ups.

The previous three cohorts all followed the same survey design: a systematic random sample with the cohort members being identified at birth as having a birthday in the chosen week of the 52 possible weeks in the year. The Millennium Cohort had a new sample design as it was both clustered and disproportionately stratified. The MCS sample consists of all children who were living in a selected electoral ward at the age of nine months. The primary sampling unit (or cluster) is the electoral ward. These wards were divided into those with a high proportion of child poverty, those with a high proportion of ethnic minority inhabitants, and others. From these three strata the electoral wards were chosen randomly, over sampling from the areas with a high proportion of child poverty, high proportion of ethnic minority inhabitants, and the Celtic countries (Plewis *et al.* 2004b).

An additional benefit of this sample design is that it ensures these subsamples are of a sufficient size, through time. This is because those over sampled – largely those who are disadvantaged or from an ethnic minority – are more likely to attrite from the sample with time. Over sampling at the start should ensure sufficient sample for future, as well as initial, analysis. One weakness in this design is that it identifies those who are disadvantaged or from ethnic minority background groups as those who live in areas with others from a similar background, but it is less likely to find people who are equally part of these groups but do not live in areas with similar people. This can be seen in the make up of the total sample with regard to ethnicity as the MCS has identified a large number of people who are identified as Pakistani or Bangladeshi but not as many in other ethnic minority groups (e.g. Chinese). This may be because those of Pakistani or Bangladeshi origin are more likely to live in areas with more homogeneous populations than the other ethnic minority groups.

Second, this design enables the Millennium Cohort Study to include all those born across an entire year of births rather than across a week of births. This enables the consideration of season of birth variation in outcomes of interest.

Third, a very large benefit of the Millennium Cohort Study is that it is focused much more broadly than the previous cohort studies. The earlier cohort studies have been largely medically focused, especially in the early years of the studies (although they have been extended to consider other economic and social outcomes in the adult years) (Ferri *et al.* 2003). In contrast, the Millennium Cohort Study has been multidisciplinary from the first sweep (Dex and Joshi 2005). The Millennium Cohort Study is therefore more suited than its predecessors to research regarding the understanding of family, community, and social change on socio-economic as well as health outcomes. This is because the Millennium Cohort Study collects a wider range of data from the first sweep about the child, their family, and their community/area in which they live.

Fourth, the data on the community/area collected directly from the participants can be enhanced through data linkage. The cluster design of the survey enables data to be added from the census and other sources at the electoral ward level. For example, in this chapter I shall present some results from having added to the data regional and local unemployment rates from external data for the area the individual was living in. In addition to data enhancement by electoral ward/region, the MCS data has also been enhanced at the individual level by linking in data from birth registrations and hospital episodes data.

Overall, the Millennium Cohort Study can be used to consider individual, family, community, and social change in various ways. It is an extensive quantitative longitudinal study. The fact that it is longitudinal enables the researcher to consider changes over the life course of the studies' participants. In addition, the fact that the MCS is one of four national cohort studies allows comparisons across the generations represented in the studies. Finally, the survey design of the MCS, which is different from the other cohorts, allows the comparison and study of various subgroups of current policy interest (e.g. the disadvantaged and ethnic minorities), as well as allowing comparisons between and within the four countries of the UK.

An example of the use of the Millennium Cohort Study: early motherhood and the family context

In this part of the chapter I present some analysis using the first two sweeps of the Millennium Cohort Study as an illustration of the potential use of this data for the study of individual, family, community, and social change. At the time of writing only data from the first two sweeps of data was available and therefore the opportunity to consider the changes over the life course is limited. I present here the starting point for the children of the Millennium Cohort Study in terms of their mothers' life experience to date, and point to how future data collection may be used to consider how these children and their families evolve over time. This particular example uses the second survey for some additional retrospective information about the family of origin of the survey child's mother, not the follow-up information about circumstances when the child reached the age of three.

This chapter expands on the analysis of the first survey (Hawkes *et al.* 2004). The topic of interest is the age at which the cohort child's mother had her first child, and how far it can be predicted by features of the woman's family of origin and her own childhood, on the one hand, and the state of the labour market around the time of conception on the other. The hypothesis in the first set of relationships is that women with a more advantaged background may have more reason to delay motherhood (both to complete education and establish careers), although features of individual families' or community culture may also have a detectable influence. Second, the state of the labour market could affect the timing of motherhood in either direction: a shortage of jobs could make early motherhood look like an attractive alternative to unemployment without a family role, or it could delay decisions to set up home until at least one partner has a job.

I consider some of the possible correlates of the age at motherhood from the early life experience of the mothers of the cohort members. These early life experiences of the cohort child's mother are likely to feed through into the early life experience of the cohort child themselves, in the form, for example, of parenting styles and the mother's expectations for her child. This analysis estimates the following equation:

$$agemoth = \alpha + \beta\ antecedent + \gamma\ labourmarket + \varepsilon$$

where *agemoth* is a continuous variable of the age at first birth or motherhood; α is the constant; *antecedent* is a set of variables which are determined before the birth of the child; *labourmarket* is those variables which consider the health of the economy, national or local, in the year before their first birth; and ε is the residual. As the dependent variable is continuous I estimate these models using an OLS regression analysis.

As the MCS dataset focuses on the cohort child itself, the current family context, and wider environment, there is relatively little information on the early life experience of the cohort member's mother. The antecedent variables observed at sweep one (when the cohort child is nine months old) consist of the mother's ethnic group (recorded as seven dummy variables), whether her parents separated or divorced before the birth of the mother's first child, and whether she had experienced any time in care as a child. In addition, a variable is derived to represent whether or not the mother left school at the compulsory school leaving age of 16 (or 15 for the few women born before 1958) as antecedent, even though in a few cases motherhood may have preceded school leaving. This variable may not be as appropriate to those who have undertaken their education outside of the UK as to those who were educated in the UK. Nonetheless, it does still provide a measure of attendance in education after the age of 16 (or 15) for all.

The earlier work (Hawkes *et al.* 2004) is extended in two ways. First, retrospective data from sweep two is included: whether the mother was born in the UK, if her parents were born in the UK, and whether her parents were employed when she was 14 years old. Additional data regarding the classification of these parental occupations will be available in the future but the coding of this data was not available in time for this study.

Second, measures of ward non-participation (or economic inactivity) as well as regional and national unemployment rates (lagged one year) are included. These data were obtained from the Office for National Statistics and based on estimates using the Labour Force Survey. Before 1992 this was an annual survey. The Labour Force Survey became quarterly in 1992; since then the spring quarter of each year has been taken. The unemployment data has been used in two ways. First, when considering all of the MCS mothers I have a group of women who became mothers between 1969 and 2002. For this set of analyses, presented in Table 10.1, lagged national unemployment rates are used. This is to represent the national economy picture at the time around the conception of the first child. Second, for those mothers for whom the cohort child is their first-born child, it is possible to identify where they were living around the time of the conception of the cohort child. Therefore, for this sub-sample (around 50 per cent of the cohort) we are able to use measures of regional unemployment as presented in Table 10.2 (that is the nine regions of England, Wales, Scotland, and Northern Ireland) as well as measures of ward-level non-participation as presented in Table 10.3. The non-participation rate is defined as the reverse of the employment rate (economic inactivity including unemployment or non-employment rate among all adults).

Appendix 1 contains the descriptive statistics of these variables used in the analyses below. The average age at first birth for all the mothers analysed was 25.7 years. For the subset of mothers whose cohort child was the first born (in 2000–2002) the average age was somewhat older at 27.0 years, reflecting the general trend away from early motherhood in the previous three decades. The average unemployment rate at the year preceding the first birth was higher for the whole sample (whose first births were spread between 1969 and 2002) than for the subset (whose cohort child was born in 2000–2002). Weighted by the number of mothers having their first child in each year, the average unemployment rate for the whole sample was 7.2 per cent, whereas the average unemployment rate in the year before the cohort children were born was 5.8 per cent.

Table 10.1 presents the results of estimating the above equation for all natural mothers in the Millennium Cohort Study. In the first column, the age at first motherhood is associated with just the antecedent variables identified at sweep one of the MCS. In all cases a negative coefficient shows that the older the mother is at the birth of her first child the less likely she is to have experienced the characteristic displayed; a positive coefficient shows an older mother is more likely to have experienced this characteristic. Therefore, those who enter motherhood later are less likely to have experienced the separation of their own parents, less likely to have experienced life in care, less likely to have left school at the minimum school leaving age, and less likely to be from an ethnic minority group (especially of Pakistani or Bangladeshi origin), relative to the white group. Another way of putting this is that staying on at school raises the average age of motherhood by over three years

Table 10.1 Regression analysis of age at first motherhood for all MCS mothers

	Mother characteristics at MCS1 (1)	Adding national unemployment rate (2)	Adding mother characteristics at MCS2 (3)
Parents separated/divorced before first birth	−1.876− (17.22)**	−1.950 (18.41)**	−1.620 (12.77)**
Ever in care at some point in childhood	−3.157 (7.39)**	−2.883 (7.07)**	−3.223 (5.90)**
Left school at the compulsory leaving age	−3.755 (25.17)**	3.459 (24.74)**	−3.099 (22.21)**
Ethnicity (reference category white)			
Mixed	−1.533 (3.46)**	−1.444 (3.39)**	−2.273 (3.66)**
Indian	−1.615 (4.89)**	−1.531 (4.72)**	−2.990 (6.92)**
Pakistani	−3.235 (14.45)**	−3.229 (15.77)**	−4.636 (13.55)**
Bangladeshi	−4.926 (24.36)**	−4.875 (25.34)**	−5.955 (18.63)**
Black Caribbean	−1.081 (1.99)*	−0.799 (1.56)	−1.194 (1.65)
Black African	−0.668 (1.75)	−0.345 (0.83)	−1.415 (2.68)**
Other ethnic group	−0.102 (0.27)	−0.231 (0.61)	−1.389 (2.93)**
Lagged national unemployment rate		−0.644 (23.87)**	0.715 (23.07)**−
Born in the UK			−0.112 (0.44)
Mother born in the UK			−0.807 (2.99)**
Father born in the UK			−0.574 (2.05)*
Mother worked when respondent 14			−0.071 (0.59)
Father worked when respondent 14			2.410 (11.49)**

continued

Table 10.1 continued Regression analysis of age at first motherhood for all MCS mothers

	Mother characteristics at MCS 1 (1)	Adding national unemployment rate (2)	Adding mother characteristics at mcs2 (3)
Constant	28.238	32.776	32.565
	(189.09)**	(112.76)**	(70.33)**
Observations	18671	18671	12905
R-squared	0.17	0.20	0.22

Notes: Absolute value of t statistics in parentheses * significant at 5%; ** significant at 1%

compared to those who left at the minimum age; having experienced family break-up lowers the average age by nearly two years; and the age at motherhood of Bangladeshi women, other things being equal, is around five years younger than white mothers.

The second column includes the lagged national unemployment rate, which is the national unemployment rate just before the time of conception. This shows that higher national unemployment rates are associated with the cohort mothers being younger at the time of their first birth. That is, a 1 per cent point increase in the national unemployment rate lowers the average age of first births to these women by 0.644 years (7.7 months). This estimate is generated from evidence over several decades and may carry within it other trended factors.

The third column adds the antecedent variables identified retrospectively at sweep two of the MCS. Note that the sample size is reduced largely due to the attrition between the first and the second sweeps of the MCS. This shows that those with parents who were born outside of the UK are, other things such as ethnic group and education being equal, less likely to be younger mothers; this is a bit surprising as migration status was expected to mediate ethnic differences rather than increase them. In addition, it shows that those with an employed father at age 14 are more likely to be older mothers at the time of their first birth.

Overall, Table 10.1 shows that mothers who entered motherhood earlier are more likely to have experienced family disruption in their own childhood, left school early, belong to ethnic minorities, and have had an unemployed father at the age of 14. Earlier motherhood is linked to earlier family disadvantage, as expected, and, in this model, to lower prospects in the national labour market. Earlier motherhood is not linked to international immigration once ethnic group is controlled.

The weakness of these results is that the national unemployment rate may not represent the state of the labour market locally facing the mother at the time of conception. Therefore, Table 10.2 uses regional rather than national unemployment rates. To do this the analysis sample has to be restricted to those cohort members who are the first born in their family because we know approximately where the mother was living at the time of conception. Table 10.2 presents these results. Again in the first column, the age at first motherhood is associated with just the antecedent variables identified at sweep one of the MCS. The results produce the same pattern to those in Table 10.1.

Table 10.2 Regression analysis of age at motherhood and regional unemployment rate: MCS mothers whose cohort child is their first

	Mother characteristics at MCS1	Adding regional unemployment	Adding area characteristics	Adding mother characteristics at MCS2
	(1)	(2)	(3)	(4)
Parents separated/divorced before first birth	−2.387 (13.63)**	−2.394 (13.61)**	−2.196 (12.57)**	−1.834 (9.13)**
Ever in care at some point in childhood	−2.690 (4.28)**	−2.700 (4.29)**	−2.218 (3.81)**	−2.531 (2.66)**
Left school at the compulsory leaving age	−3.336 (16.09)**	−3.328 (15.75)**	−2.981 (14.63)**	−2.648 (12.22)**
Ethnicity (reference category white)	−1.507		−1.173	−1.748
Mixed	−1.642 (2.23)*	−1.657 (2.25)*	−1.378 (1.96)	−1.690 (2.02)*
Indian	−1.462 (3.04)**	−1.425 (2.91)**	−1.013 (2.25)*	−3.524 (5.34)**
Pakistani	−4.122 (10.23)**	−4.109 (10.14)**	−3.091 (7.61)**	−5.125 (8.71)**
Bangladeshi	−5.184 (13.08)**	−5.112 (12.64)**	−4.266 (8.04)**	−6.013 (7.61)**
Black Caribbean	−0.225 (0.27)	−0.156 (0.18)	0.389 (0.47)	0.499 (0.42)
Black African	0.007 (0.01)	0.084 (0.12)	0.835 (1.08)	−1.544 (1.47)
Other ethnic group	0.497 (0.86)	0.557 (0.96)	0.841 (1.55)	−1.167 (1.65)
Regional unemployment rate		−0.066 (0.69)	0.156 (1.56)	0.131 (1.35)
Country (reference England)				
Wales			−1.257 (3.94)**	0.977 (3.18)**

continued

Table 10.2 continued Regression analysis of age at motherhood and regional unemployment rate: MCS mothers whose cohort child is their first

	Mother characteristics at MCS1	Adding Regional unemployment	Adding area characteristics	Adding mother characteristics at MCS2
	(1)	(2)	(3)	(4)
Scotland			−0.543 (1.39)	−0.036 (0.08)
Northern Ireland			−1.513 (4.49)**	−1.572 (4.36)**
Area type				
Disadvantaged			−2.353 (8.58)**	−2.044 (7.38)**
Ethnic			−2.448 (5.51)**	−2.507 (5.23)**
Born in the UK				−0.871 (2.34)*
Mother born in the UK				−1.229 (3.02)**
Father born in the UK				−0.816 (1.81)
Mother worked when respondent 14				0.247 −(1.24)
Father worked when respondent 14				2.393 (6.59)**
Constant	29.235 (170.71)**	29.618 (54.04)**	29.143 (51.94)**	29.886 (39.93)**
Observations	7658	7658	7658	5323
R−squared	0.14	0.14	0.17	0.18

Notes: Absolute value of t statistics in parentheses * significant at 5%; ** significant at 1%

In the second column, the regional unemployment rate is included. While it is insignificant, and of much smaller magnitude, it is of the same sign as the national unemployment rate in Table 10.1. In the third column, including some area characteristics, the regional unemployment rate changes sign from a negative to a positive, but still has no significant association. However, living in areas of high child poverty ('disadvantaged' area type) or in areas with high proportions of ethnic minorities (which are also areas of high unemployment rates) is associated with younger mothers. In addition, living in Wales and Northern Ireland is associated with younger mothers relative to England.

When the antecedent variables from sweep two are included, regional unemployment remains insignificantly positive. However, it is strongly outweighed by the area characteristics (which are probably a better measure of the local labour market). Once again, having a UK-born parent means that, all else such as school leaving being equal, the mother is more likely to have had her first child younger. Older mothers are more likely to have fathers who were employed when they were 14 years old.

Overall, Table 10.2 shows patterns similar to Table 10.1: the younger mothers of first-born children in the cohort are more likely to have experienced disadvantaged backgrounds themselves. In addition, the children of younger mothers are more likely to be born in a disadvantaged area (an area with higher rates of child poverty and higher proportion of ethnic minorities). In the final two columns the sign of the coefficient on the regional unemployment variable becomes positive. Therefore, regional unemployment appears to delay motherhood, provided there is not a family history of worklessness or the mother is not living in a particularly disadvantaged area. The regional unemployment rate does not appear to be disaggregated enough to really represent the state of the labour market locally that is experienced by the mother at the time of conception. Therefore, Table 10.3 uses ward-level non-participation rates rather than national unemployment rates.

Table 10.3 Regression analysis of age at first motherhood for first born: MCS mothers and ward-level non-participation rates

	Mother characteristics at MCS1	Adding area characteristics	Adding ward non-participation	Adding mother characteristics at MCS2
	(1)	(2)	(3)	(4)
Parents separated/divorced before first birth	−2.387 (13.63)**	−2.419 (13.94)**	−2.213 (12.90)**	−1.860 (9.39)**
Ever in care at some point in childhood	−2.690 (4.28)**	−2.690 (4.25)**	−2.273 (3.81)**	−2.644 (2.78)**
Left school at the compulsory leaving age	−3.336 (16.09)**	−3.332 (16.30)**	−2.969 (14.20)**	−2.645 (12.02)**
Ethnicity (reference category white)				
Mixed	−1.642 (2.23)*	−1.766 (2.41)*	−1.415 (1.99)*	−1.745 (2.11)*

continued

Table 10.3 continued Regression analysis of age at first motherhood for first born: MCS mothers and ward-level non-participation rates

	Mother characteristics at MCS1	Adding area characteristics	Adding ward non-participation	Adding mother characteristics at MCS2
	(1)	(2)	(3)	(4)
Indian	−1.462 (3.04)**	−1.592 (3.34)**	−0.979 (2.20)*	−3.463 (5.28)**
Pakistani	−4.122 (10.23)**	−4.221 (10.42)**	−3.087 (7.16)**	−5.128 (8.32)**
Bangladeshi	−5.184 (13.08)**	−5.212 (13.22)**	−3.899 (7.51)**	−5.649 (7.12)**
Black Caribbean	−0.225 (0.27)	−0.280 (0.33)	0.609 (0.74)	0.693 (0.59)
Black African	0.007 (0.01)	−0.077 (0.11)	1.102 (1.47)	−1.351 (1.32)
Other ethnic group	0.497 (0.86)	0.445 (0.77)	1.006 (1.90)	−1.085 (1.54)
Ward non-participation rate		−0.014 (4.01)**	−0.044 (2.82)**	−0.037 (2.36)*
Country (reference England)				
Wales			−0.657 (1.94)	−0.473 (1.45)
Scotland			3.170 (2.48)*	3.135 (2.41)*
Northern Ireland			2.116 (1.67)	1.516 (1.18)
Area type				
Disadvantaged			−2.050 (7.49)**	−1.786 (6.54)**
Ethnic			−1.935 (4.24)**	−2.101 (4.28)**
Born in the UK				−0.854 (2.24)*
Mother born in the UK				−1.201 (2.96)**
Father born in the UK				−0.860 (1.89)
Mother worked when respondent 14				−0.277 (1.38)
Father worked when respondent 14				2.322 (6.37)**

continued

Table 10.3 continued Regression analysis of age at first motherhood for first born: MCS mothers and ward-level non-participation rates

	Mother characteristics at MCS1	Adding area characteristics	Adding ward non-participation	Adding mother characteristics at MCS2
	(1)	(2)	(3)	(4)
Constant	29.235	29.722	30.922	31.473
	(170.71)**	(129.20)**	(82.39)**	(46.72)**
Observations	7658	7658	7658	5323
R-squared	0.14	0.14	0.18	0.18

Notes: Absolute value of t statistics in parentheses * significant at 5%; ** significant at 1%

Table 10.3 follows a structure similar to Table 10.2 as the same is once again restricted to mothers whose cohort child is their first born. The first column is the same as in Table 10.2. In the second column the inclusion of ward non-participation rate is significantly negative. A 1 per cent increase in ward non-participation reduces the average age of motherhood by 0.014 years or 0.168 months. This suggests that children of younger mothers are more likely to be born in electoral wards with higher non-participation rates. Including the area characteristics in the third column again shows that those born to younger mothers are more likely to have been born in areas with higher levels of child poverty and higher proportions of ethnic minorities. However, the inclusion of the ward-level non-participation rates rather than regional unemployment changes the country effects with Scotland now having, all else being equal, significantly older mothers than the rest of the UK. Finally, the inclusion of the antecedent variables recorded at the second sweep of MCS again shows that those who have parents born inside of the UK and workless fathers at age 14 are, all else being equal, likely to be younger at the time of their first birth. The addition of terms in the third and fourth columns of Table 10.3 does not reduce the negative estimate for ward non-participation rates as it did for regional unemployment in Table 10.2; if anything, it strengthens the rather small negative association of non-participation rate and early motherhood.

Overall, Table 10.3 confirms the association of early motherhood and antecedent and contemporaneous disadvantages. In addition, Table 10.3 provides evidence that the local employment prospects appear to encourage delayed motherhood where they are good, and earlier childbearing where the alternatives to it are not so good. From this it is possible to conclude that those born to younger parents are more likely to be exposed to the disadvantages from their mother's background as well as those of living in a more disadvantaged area.

How do these results relate to the study of individual, family, community, and social change?

First, MCS children who were born to mothers who were in their teens and early twenties when they had their first child, tended to have mothers who had experienced tougher childhoods themselves and to be more likely to be raised in disadvantaged areas. Hawkes and colleagues (2004) find that these antecedent disadvantages are compounded by poorer circumstances in which the cohort children find themselves at sweep one. Early motherhood (including mothers in their mid-twenties, not just teens), is a marker for prospective disadvantage and itself reflects a cycle of disadvantage preceding it and following the event. As the MCS continues it will be possible to see how these differences in family background will be associated with future socio-economic and health outcomes. This is of particular policy interest as in the past ten years child poverty and area regeneration have become an important part of the government's targets. This means that the Millennium Cohort Study is well-placed as a data set in time to see if these policy initiatives have been successful.

Second, while not discussed here, with time it will be possible to compare the life courses of these children with the older cohorts. It is possible that, with the growth of female employment and education, this cohort has a much more polarised distribution of age of mother than the previous cohorts. This could be related to differential life chances for those born to younger mothers today than in the past. It will be possible to address such questions by the MCS and its family of cohort studies in the future. It is a challenge to the research community to exploit this new resource.

Note

1 I would like to thank the Economic and Social Research Council for funding this research (grant number RES-163-25-0002). A special thanks to Heather Joshi for all her helpful comments and suggestions on the previous version of the paper that led to this chapter. Finally I would like to thank Mark Killingsworth, Constantinos Kallis, Fiona Steele and the participants at: the British Society for Population Studies Conference in Canterbury 2005, the XIX Annual Conference of the European Society for Population Economics in Paris 2005, and the ESRC seminar series on Family, Community and Social Change 2005 for their comments and suggestions. All remaining errors are my own.

References

Brassett-Grundy, A., Joshi, H. and Butler, N. (2004) 'Millennium Cohort Study: Health Visitor Survey Interim Report', February, London: Centre for Longitudinal Studies.

Bynner, J. (2004) 'Longitudinal Cohort Designs' in K. Kempf-Leonard (ed.) *Encyclopaedia of Social Measurement,* vol 2, San Diego: Elsevier.

Dex, S. and Joshi, H. (2005) *Children of the 21st Century: From Birth to Nine Months,* Bristol: The Policy Press.

Ferri, E., Bynner, J. and Wadsworth, M. (eds) (2003) *Changing Britain, Changing Lives: Three Generations at the Turn of the Century,* London: Bedford Way Papers, Institute of Education.

Hansen, K. (2006) *Millennium Cohort Study First and Second Survey: A Guide to the Datasets,* London: Centre for Longitudinal Studies.

Hawkes, D. and Plewis, I. (2006) 'Modelling Non-Response in the National Child Development Survey', *Journal of the Royal Statistical Society Series A (Statistics in Society),* July, vol. 169, 479–93.

Hawkes, D., Joshi, H. and Ward, K. (2004) 'Unequal Entry to Motherhood and Unequal Starts in Life: Evidence from the First Survey of the UK Millennium Cohort', CLS Working Paper, London: Centre for Longitudinal Studies.

Plewis, I., Calderwood, L., Hawkes, D. and Nathan, G. (2004a) *National Child Development Study and 1970 British Cohort Study Technical Report: Changes in the NCDS and BCS70 Populations and Samples over Time,* London: Centre for Longitudinal Studies.

Plewis, I., Calderwood, L., Hawkes, D., Hughes, G. and Joshi, H. (2004b) *Millennium Cohort Study First Survey: Technical Report on Sampling,* Third Edition, London: Centre for Longitudinal Studies.

Shepherd, P. (1995) 'The National Child Development Study (NCDS): An Introduction to the Origins of the Study and the Methods of Data Collection', *NCDS User Support Group* Working Paper 1 (Revised), London: Social Statistics Research Unit, City University.

Wadsworth, M. E. J. (1991) *The Imprint of Time,* Oxford: Oxford University Press.

Appendix I Descriptive statistics

	National unemployment (Table 10.1) (1)	Regional unemployment (Table 10.2) (2)	Ward unemployment (Table 10.3) (3)
Mother's age at first birth	25.70 (0.14)	27.02 (0.17)	27.02 (0.17)
MCS1 mother characteristics			
Parents separated/divorced before first birth	0.28	0.29	0.29
Ever in care at some point in childhood	0.01	0.01	0.01
Left school at the compulsory leaving age	0.46	0.41	0.41

continued

Appendix I continued Descriptive statistics

	National unemployment (Table 10.1) (1)	Regional unemployment (Table 10.2) (2)	Ward unemployment (Table 10.3) (3)
Ethnicity			
White	0.89	0.90	0.90
Mixed	0.01	0.01	0.01
Indian	0.02	0.02	0.02
Pakistani	0.03	0.02	0.02
Bangladeshi	0.01	0.01	0.01
Black Caribbean	0.01	0.01	0.01
Black African	0.01	0.01	0.01
Other ethnic group	0.02	0.02	0.02
Labour market			
Unemployment/ non-participation rate %	7.25 (0.02)	5.84 (0.11)	34.6* (0.68)
Area Characteristics			
Country			
England		0.82	0.82
Wales		0.05	0.05
Scotland		0.10	0.10
Northern Ireland		0.03	0.03
Area Type			
Advantaged		0.61	0.61
Disadvantaged		0.35	0.35
Ethnic		0.04	0.04
MCS2 mother characteristics			
Born in the UK	0.90	0.92	0.92
Mother born in the UK	0.85	0.87	0.87
Father born in the UK	0.84	0.87	0.87
Mother worked when respondent 14	0.69	0.71	0.71
Father worked when respondent 14	0.93	0.93	0.93
Unweighted observations	18671	7658	5323

Notes: Weighted proportions or weighted means with adjusted standard errors in parentheses are presented. *This is the ward level non-participation rate of all adults of working age (16–64) rather than an actual unemployment rate – as the ward level unemployment rate was not available.

Chapter 11

Using longitudinal data to examine living alone in England and Wales

1971 to 2001

Malcolm Williams, Moira Maconachie, Lawrence Ware, Joan Chandler, and Brian Dodgeon

Introduction

While there has been a long-standing interest, particularly by policy-makers, in solo-living amongst the elderly, and although it is acknowledged as one of the most important demographic trends in our society, there has been less sociological work on living alone as a more general household arrangement across the life course of individuals. This chapter provides a contextual description of the patterning of living alone amongst working age people in England and Wales between 1971 and 2001.

One of the reasons for the relative absence of sociological work on living alone may be that as a living arrangement it has fallen outside analyses of and research on families. For the last quarter of a century or so sociologists have been mainly concerned with the diversity of forms family living has taken, including lone-parenting, cohabitation, step-families, and gay couples/parenting (Silva and Smart 1999). Early on, Gittins (1985) queried a notion of 'the family', maintaining that instead we should speak of 'families' as diverse kinship structures. Especially amongst younger people, sociologists have regarded living alone as 'non-family living' (Goldscheider and Waite 1991) or as indicating the rise in 'non-familial' or 'post-familial' families (Allan and Jones 2003; Beck-Gernsheim 2002). However, these characterisations ignore the relationships between people who live alone and other family members and household structures. While living alone (as we will show here) is an increasing phenomenon in an individual's life course, it has implications for the specific family or household arrangements that an individual may come from or go to, and it also has implications for families and communities more generally. Living alone does not necessarily imply an atomistic existence for the individual. For many who live alone, kinship bonds or relationships continue to exist (Roseneil and Budgeon 2004; Levin 2004). Jamieson and colleagues (2003) conducted interviews with single people in their twenties and found that over half described themselves as in a relationship.

The concept of living alone also blurs the distinction between 'family' and 'household'. Allan and Crow (2001) have noted that contemporary analyses of family life demand greater precision in the use of the terms 'family' and 'household'. They also note how difficult this precision is as the terms are used interchangeably in everyday life and frequently within sociology. Relationships and living arrangements are often conflated and analysts frequently have to read between the lines. Living alone is an ambiguous concept and may incorporate a range of different kinds of living arrangements and kinship and friendship relationships.

The growth and prominence of living alone

The increase in the numbers of persons living alone has constituted one of the most profound demographic changes in Britain, and in Europe more generally, in the last 30 years (Kaufmann 1994). While the population of Great Britain has grown by 5 per cent over the past three decades, the number of households with one occupant has grown by 31 per cent (Office for National Statistics 2003: 42). The 2001 Census indicated that 16 per cent of all adults under pensionable age were living alone.

An emergent trend in the social patterning of solo living is that those who live alone are younger, increasingly male, amongst the younger age groups, urban, and professional. Also, an increasing proportion of those who live alone have moved away from the private rented accommodation that was once associated with this group, to become owner-occupiers. A survey of the housing preferences of those who lived alone in the early 1990s found that over the life course they shared similar housing preferences and aspirations to couple and family households (Strode 1998; Hooper *et al.* 1998).

The rise of solo living is frequently seen as an indicator of 'individualisation'. Beck-Gernsheim (2002), for example, argues that the greater choice and the greater fragility of contemporary relationships means that lone occupant households are more likely to occur throughout an adult's life and have different implications and meanings at different points. Furthermore, Bawin-Legros' analysis (2001, 2004) of the new sentimental order emphasised the reformation of intimacy values and their implications for interdependencies. This interplays with living arrangements as people's reference points shift from collectives to the individual and from an obligation to others to their freedom to choose and their right to privacy.

The work of social theorists (Giddens 1992; Beck and Beck-Gernsheim 1995, 2002; Bauman 2003) has raised important issues about the causes and effects of living alone for society. These effects, if demonstrated, will have important implications for emotional relationships and the nature of household formation and dissolution, but also on the resource needs (such as housing and care) in society. Yet much of this work, however persuasive or plausible, is at the level of theory. Furthermore, while there has been a plethora of sociological research on the changing nature of families, alternative manifestations of relationships and friendships/ friendship networks, there has been little research on the characteristics of living alone over the life course. National population data have demonstrated the trend toward living alone and provided descriptions of the age and sex of those who live alone but, until recently, there was little numeric data on the transitions into and out of such living arrangements. More specifically: what were the prior household arrangements of those who come to live alone?; did previous household arrangements vary by age or sex?; and once living alone, were people more likely to remain in that state?

Measuring household change using census data

The research reported in this chapter draws upon a life course framework, comparing the changing pattern of household transformation between different age groups (Giele and Elder 1998). It provides an overview of the shift to living alone over time and through people's lives, but more generally it provides a structural context for further sociological or policy-related research on communities and the family. Indeed its main purpose is to provide a methodological discussion of the usefulness and limitations of longitudinal statistical data on living alone.

Our data source (the Longitudinal Study) is a 1 per cent sample of linked individual Census records from England and Wales for each Census from 1971 to 2001. The total sample is around 500,000 people. Initially, all people born on each of four dates in any year were selected from information given in the 1971 Census. From 1971, as new births occur on these four dates each year, the persons are added to the sample. As immigrants with those birth dates register with the National Health Service, they also join the LS. At each Census since 1971, data relating to LS members and, to some extent, members of their household, have been added. Thus the LS is a true longitudinal study, a continuous sample from 1971. The sample size remains proportional to the population, but because people leave the study through death or migration from England and Wales, the sample enumerated of those present at two or more Censuses is substantially lower than the 1 per cent sample at any one Census. Because a sample of all those present at each Census from 1971 to 2001 would be considerably smaller and would have a truncated age distribution, our research was conducted in two stages. In stage one our sample was that of all adults aged 15[1] to 44 in 1971 and enumerated at their home address at each Census from 1971 to 1991 inclusive. In stage two our sample was that of all adults aged 16 to 44 in 1981 and enumerated at their home address at each Census from 1981 to 2001 inclusive. Each sample comprises LS members of working age (over each 20-year period) which allowed us to track adult household moves, but selected out those moves made by children or the elderly.[2]

Because patterns in our second sample were very similar, though sometimes accentuated, most of the analyses presented and discussed below are based on the (second) sample of 1981–2001.

Advantages of the LS

The LS is the largest truly longitudinal data set in England and Wales[3] that can track individuals through much, or the whole of their life course. With data available for each ten-year Census from 1971 to 2001 it is possible to track the life course of individuals to show not just their household transitions, but changes in their marital status, tenure, employment, and numbers of children. Because the LS is based upon the England and Wales Census it has universal coverage with a response rate of around 98 per cent and is not geographically skewed. Even relatively small numbers will therefore be statistically significant (Hattersley and Creeser 1995).

Disadvantages of the LS

Nevertheless, there are limitations to the LS. First, it is a wholly descriptive data set, limited to Census variables, with no attitudinal data. It cannot tell us why people live alone, nor why they choose or are constrained to living in subsequent household arrangements – though analyses of household movements combined with other variables can provide important clues to behaviour and circumstances. However, it must be made clear that the purpose of the research was to map household transitions that might provide a useful basis for attitudinal or detailed behavioural research.

Second, though the data are truly longitudinal – the same individuals are followed through time and the Census points are 'snapshots' – an LS member may be enumerated in the same household arrangement at two consecutive Censuses, but they may have lived in other arrangements in the period between and intermediate household transitions are not recorded. Nevertheless, it seems a reasonable assumption that within the sample such a diversity of intermediate states would cancel each other out to some extent.

Third, the difficulties of delay and standardisation should be noted, though these are not serious problems. Delay refers to the time lapse between the Census and the availability of LS data. Fortunately, the phenomenon of living alone has exhibited rather similar trends over time and delay factor is somewhat off-set by its longevity. The trends we report here have been observed, in a longitudinal sample, over 30 years. Similarly, standardisation, though not an insignificant technical issue, does not impinge on validity and reliability. The principle dependent variable in this study – household structure – is derived from slightly different measures at each Census. The residual category of 'other' describes those cases that cannot be attributed to other household structures and arise mainly as a result of the standardisation procedure.

What is meant by 'living alone' and how did we measure it?

As a sociological category, living alone is far from simple: it is not a dichotomous state of living alone or not living alone. People's daily household arrangements do not conform to such simple patterns. A person who 'lives alone' may have a partner or other relative who spends time with them. Their level of other kinds of friendship or social interaction may vary considerably and change character over quite short periods of time. Relationships and living arrangements are often ambiguously reported and the nature of living arrangements must be subject to some interpretation and imputation. For example, the boundaries between living alone and cohabitation are blurred and some care is required in the use of the terms 'family' and 'household' (Allan and Crow 2001). Nevertheless, a limitation of population data is inevitably the need to simplify and use fixed operationalisable terms to produce reliable measures over time (Williams 2003).

In the analyses presented in this chapter we were constrained to using a Census-derived definition of living alone that depends on the respondent's self-declared status on Census night. Though this definition could obscure a number of variations of living arrangements, because they are consistently measured over time they do have reliability and longitudinal validity (Collett *et al.* 2006).

The LS category of 'living alone' is one of 12 household types originally derived by Overton and Ermisch (1984) and developed for the LS by Williams and Dale (1991) and Dale *et al.* (1996). Because our analyses excluded elderly persons (of 65 years or older) and some household type categories were very small, it was possible to use a simplified nine-category typology:

- One person living alone
- Non-married adults
- Married couple
    no children
    dependent children
    dependent children and others
    non-dependent or others
- Lone parents
- Complex households
- Others.

These household structure types represent the logical possibilities of household arrangements of adults and children. Some of these provide indicators of marriage, cohabiting, and childrearing arrangements, thus an exit from a household characterised as a married couple with children to living alone, is an indication of a relationship breakdown in most cases. However, some caution is needed here because amongst younger people (in our age categorisation 16–24 year olds), the person who subsequently leaves this arrangement may be a dependent child who is now an adult and has left the family home. Indeed this holds true for other groups. For example, a move from a lone parent family to living alone amongst the older age groups indicates that this is the parent and the child has grown up and left, but amongst the younger age group the person living alone is almost certainly the son or daughter.

The growth and stability of living alone 1971–2001

LS data allows us to both follow people in different age cohorts, as they grow older and to track whether they enter, remain in or leave lone-person households. So, for example, we can take those who were aged 15 to 24 in 1971 and look at the kind of household they lived in at subsequent Censuses. Additionally we can take age bands at each Census and compare them cross-sectionally to measure whether people in those age bands at each Census are more or less likely to live alone. In Table 1 we have joined together our two samples to show the general pattern in living alone over time.

By following the diagonal line of each age band it is possible to see how living alone increases across the life course of the sample members. For example, 1.9 per cent of 16–24 year olds lived alone in 1981, but as this cohort aged they were more likely to live alone; by 2001 9.0 per cent of them lived in this household category. The nature of the samples means that we do not have data on the youngest age band in later Censuses, or the older ones in earlier Censuses, but nevertheless by following the horizontal line of each age band we can see the growth in living alone over time. Data for 1971 in Table 11.1 is taken from the first sample (1971–1991). There were 1.1 per cent of 15–24 year olds living alone in 1971 compared to 1.9 per cent of 16–24 year olds in

Table 11.1 Percentage living alone 1971–2001 by age at Census year

Age in Census year	1971	1981	1991	2001
15–24	1.1	1.9		
25–34	1.8	3.9	7.5	
35–44	2.0	2.9	5.4	9.0
44–54		4.8	6.7	10.2
55–64			13.2	14.2

Source: ONS Longitudinal Study

1981 (our second sample). There were 2.0 per cent of 35–44 year olds living alone in 1971 and by 2001 this had increased to 9.0 per cent, indicating a rising trend over time. The total numbers living alone have grown at each Census (following the horizontal lines across the table), but also the chances of living alone have increased for people through their life course (comparing the diagonal lines down the table).

Household structure and the move to living alone

The increase in living alone in England and Wales is reflected in changes of household structure within the sample. Table 11.2 shows the proportion of the entire sample in each household structure from 1981 to 2001. The proportion of the sample living alone increased steadily over the period. In 1981 only 2.9 per cent of the sample lived alone. By 1991 the proportion living alone had increased to 6.5 per cent and by 2001 the figure was 11.2 per cent (an increase of just under 5 percentage points between each census). The increase in living alone continues the pattern observed between 1971 and 1991 (Chandler *et al.* 2004). Though living alone is the most important trend over time, lone-person households were not the only household structure that increased proportionately in the sample over the period. The proportion of the sample living as a couple with no dependent children also increased significantly. In 1981, around a tenth (10.7 per cent) of the sample lived in a 'couple with no dependent children' household. This figure increased to almost a fifth (18.4 per cent) by 1991, and by 2001 over a quarter (28.2 per cent) of the

Table 11.2 Household structure of sample 1981–2001

| Household structure | Census year/ (Age of sample) | | |
	1981 (16–44)	1991 (26–54)	2001 (36–64)
One person < 65	2.9	6.5	11.2
2+ adults, no elderly	6.3	4.0	3.2
Couple, no dependent children	10.7	18.4	28.2
Couple + dependent children	41.8	37.4	23.7
Couple + dependent children + adult	15.7	9.5	7.0
Couple, no dependent children + adult	10.4	13.8	13.6
One-parent family	6.0	4.2	3.8
Complex household	5.1	5.4	5.5
Other	1.1	0.7	3.9
Total	*100.0*	*100.0*	*100.0*
All	*162,393*	*162,393*	*162,393*

Source: ONS Longitudinal Study

sample lived within this household arrangement. Increases in this household arrangement reflect anticipated life course changes over time as a result of children leaving home. Similarly, changes in the percentages of people living in other household arrangements can be explained by this or by their becoming adults and remaining in the parental household. Living alone, by contrast, is a household form with several different kinds of routes in from other household arrangements and is more likely to occur at different points in the life course of individuals. It is these issues we now explore using longitudinal data.

Tables 11.3 and 11.4 allow us to examine the differences in life course transitions to living alone amongst men and women between 1981 and 1991 and between 1991 and 2001. Table 11.3 shows the household origins of those living alone in 1991, while Table 11.4 shows the household origins of those living alone in 2001. First, we examine the continuity of living alone from one Census point to the next; second, we explore transitions from other household structures to living alone.

The continuity of living alone 1981–2001

What is noteworthy in both these tables is the consistency of the pattern of living alone in one Census and still living alone at the next Census: Table 11.3 reveals that 16.6 per cent of all those who lived alone in 1991 had lived alone in 1981; Table 11.4 shows that 32.4 per cent of all those who were living alone in 2001 had lived alone in 1991. For both men and women, on the whole, this tendency increases in each age band and over time. Moreover comparing the tables highlights the increase in living alone for the whole sample over time: the total number of people living alone rose from 10,500 (1981–91) to just over 18,000 (1991–2001). One important difference between the two tables is that between 1981 and 1991 more people started or continued to live alone, but in the decade later proportionately fewer people moved to living alone from other household structures. However, in 2001 more of the people who had lived alone continued in this arrangement. This indicates the relative stability of living alone among older people: 35.6 per cent of men and 29.2 per cent of women who lived alone in 2001 had lived alone in 1991 (see fourth and eighth columns Table 11.4), double the percentages for 1981–91 (17.0 per cent and 15.9 per cent, respectively).

Amongst the youngest age band (26–34 years old in 1991) in Table 11.3 there is very little difference in the proportions of men (4.4 per cent) and women (4.3 per cent) that lived alone in 1981. As a household origin, living alone is small (less than 5 per cent) compared to couple households (more than 60 per cent taken altogether). This indicates that the transition to living alone (in many cases from the parental home) amongst younger people does not differ that much by sex. For those aged 35–44,[4] the percentages of men and women living alone that did so ten years earlier are also similar for both

Table 11.3 Household Structures (1981) for men and women living alone (1991) by age (%)

Household structure 1981	Age of men in 1991				Age of women in 1991				All
	26–34	35–44	45–54	All	26–34	35–44	45–54	All	
1 person < 65	4.4	23.4	28.9	17.0	4.3	25.2	19.5	15.9	16.6
2+ adults, no elderly	11.1	16.9	7.6	12.1	14.1	19.5	9.9	13.9	12.9
Couple, no dependent children	3.4	10.5	5.5	6.3	4.4	12.1	7.2	7.6	6.8
Couple + dependent children	11.0	19.1	22.4	16.7	12.7	11.8	15.9	13.7	15.4
Couple + dependent children + adult	29.3	3.7	6.4	14.9	27.4	2.8	10.7	14.1	14.6
Couple, no dependent children + adult	26.2	10.9	3.3	15.2	21.7	9.5	5.5	12.0	13.8
One-parent family	6.8	3.9	5.1	5.4	7.7	7.7	20.2	12.7	8.5
Complex household	5.4	10.0	19.6	10.6	4.3	8.5	10.0	7.7	9.4
Other	2.3	1.6	1.1	1.8	3.4	2.8	0.9	2.2	2.0
All (%)	100.0	100.0	100.0	100.0	100.0	100.0	100.0	100.0	100.0
All (N)	2,462	1,990	1,559	6,011	1,513	1,207	1,803	4,523	10,534

Source: ONS Longitudinal Study

Table 11.4 Household Structures (1991) for men and women living alone (2001) by age (%)

Household structure 1991	Age of men in 2001				Age of women in 2001				All
	36–44	45–54	55–64	All	36–44	45–54	55–64	All	
1 person < 65	30.7	37.0	39.4	35.6	30.1	26.8	30.5	29.2	32.4
2+ adults, no elderly	12.1	6.9	9.4	9.5	13.0	10.8	17.5	14.5	12.0
Couple, no dependent children	15.3	9.1	12.1	12.2	18.4	9.9	16.1	14.6	13.4
Couple + dependent children	19.2	22.1	7.7	16.6	9.5	12.9	3.9	7.9	12.2
Couple + dependent children + adult	1.6	4.9	4.8	3.7	1.7	7.0	2.7	3.9	3.8
Couple, no dependent children + adult	11.2	4.0	9.6	8.2	8.7	5.6	12.2	9.4	8.8
One-parent family	1.2	2.9	2.8	2.3	10.2	18.9	7.3	11.6	7.0
Complex household	7.7	12.1	13.4	11.0	7.0	7.3	7.5	7.3	9.2
Other	1.0	1.0	0.7	0.9	1.4	0.7	2.3	1.6	1.3
All (%)	100.0	100.0	100.0	100.0	100.0	100.0	100.0	100.0	100.0
All (N)	3,073	3,123	2,791	8,987	1,721	2,949	4,472	9,142	18,129

Source: ONS Longitudinal Study

1991 (23.4 per cent and 25.2 per cent, Table 11.3) and 2001 (30.7 per cent and 30.1 per cent, Table 11.4). In the older age bands the similarities between the proportions of men and women living alone at both points are not apparent. A total of 28.9 per cent of men aged 45–54 living alone in 1991 also did so in 1981, compared to 19.5 per cent of women (Table 11.3). Comparable differences are evident for 45–54 year olds living alone in 2001, with 37.0 per cent of these men also having done so in 1991 compared to 26.8 per cent of women (Table 11.4). The oldest age band for which we have data exhibits analogous patterns. In this age band (55–64 years old in 2001) the proportion of women living alone that also did so in 1991 is lower than for men (30.5 per cent compared to 39.4 per cent, Table 11.4).

Transitions from other household structures to living alone 1981–2001

By exploring transitions from other household arrangements to living alone we can look for evidence to account for the differences between men and women in the older age bands identified in the previous section.

Amongst the youngest age band (26–34 years old in 1991) in Table 11.3 there is very little difference in most household origins between men and women living alone.[5] There is a more noticeable difference between younger men and women that originated from 'Two adults with no elderly' households (11.1 per cent and 14.1 per cent).[6] This suggests that younger men living alone tend to leave this household arrangement earlier than young women. There is a greater difference between younger men and women originating from 'couples with dependent children and additional adult' households (29.3 per cent and 27.4 per cent). This suggests that younger men living alone are more likely than women to stay at the parental home longer in these households.

If we look at those living alone aged '35–44[7] in 2001' who moved from households characterised as 'couples with dependent children' ten years earlier, we observe clear differences between the sexes. Men this age were much more likely to have come from these households than women of the same age in both 1991 (19.1 per cent and 11.8 per cent, Table 11.3) and 2001 (19.2 per cent and 9.5 per cent, Table 11.4). These differences are also apparent for men and women living alone aged 45–54 in 1991 (22.4 per cent and 15.9 per cent, Table 11.3) and 2001 (22.1 per cent and 12.9 per cent, Table 11.4). The gender difference is almost certainly attributable to relationship breakdown and men leaving the household to live alone while the children remain in the care of their mothers (who, in contrast, tend to form lone-parent households on the breakdown of the relationship). This is substantiated by differences in later life transitions from lone-parent families to living alone for women. As many as one fifth (20.2 per cent) of women aged 45–54 living alone in

1991 (Table 11.3) came from lone-parent households while 18.9 per cent did so in 2001. For men the proportions were 5.1 per cent and 2.9 per cent, respectively. In each case these moves accounted for one of the largest percentage of household moves to living alone for women in this age band. Conversely, very few men (less than 6 per cent) that lived alone in 1991 or 2001 originated from lone-parent households.

Those people who move from 'couples plus dependent children plus other adults' and those moving from 'couples with no dependent children, but with other adults present' households to living alone, could represent several different kinds of moves. Amongst the younger age bands these are likely to be children leaving the parental home, but amongst the older bands these may well be a parent leaving the 'family' home.

We can, however, conclude that while living alone is less 'gendered' amongst younger people, there are clearer differences between the sexes in the older age bands (explained in part by women retaining responsibility for the care of children on the breakdown of couple relationships). Overall, men are more likely to live alone earlier after leaving 'couple plus children households', but for women living alone is often postponed by a period of being lone parents (Chandler *et al.* 2004; Ware *et al.* 2007).

Household structures and moves from living alone

So far we have shown that once a person lives alone they are more likely to continue to do so. In each of the Census decades since 1971, the older a person gets when they live alone, the more likely they are to remain living alone. However, we can learn a little more about the processes of living alone later in the life course by looking at exits from living alone between 1991 and 2001. There were 10,534 people living alone in 1991 (Table 11.3) and 5,874 of them continued to live alone in 2001 (32.4 per cent of 18,129, Table 11.4). We now examine the household structures of the 4,661 sample members who stopped living alone between 1991–2001. Table 11.5 shows the type of household into which those persons who lived alone in 1991, but had ceased living alone by 2001, moved.

The overall numbers moving from living alone (between 1991 and 2001) to other household structures is quite small: 4,661 in the sample or approximately 466,000 across England and Wales; 60 per cent of these were men. So while men were more likely to move into living alone, they were also more likely than women to leave this arrangement. There are also differences in the kind of exits men and women took, though there are no straightforward explanations for these differences.

Unsurprisingly, moves into couple households are the most important moves for both men and women (over 70 per cent taken altogether). A lower proportion of women moved from living alone into 'couple plus dependent children' households than men (25.7 per cent compared to 37.4 per cent),

Table 11.5 Household structures (2001) for men and women who moved from living alone (1991) by age (%)

Household structure 2001	Age of men in 1991				Age of women in 1991				All
	26–34	35–44	45–54	All	26–34	35–44	45–54	All	
2+ adults, no elderly	4.5	9.1	9.1	6.6	3.8	9.8	19.9	9.0	7.6
Couple, no dependent children	28.3	42.1	57.4	37.1	34.5	59.7	38.8	41.2	38.8
Couple + dependent children	52.3	27.4	6.7	37.4	43.8	10.0	0	25.7	32.8
Couple + dependent children + adult	4.7	4.0	1.5	4.0	1.0	0.7	1.4	1.0	2.8
Couple, no dependent children + adult	3.0	6.7	8.0	4.9	1.2	2.9	3.4	2.1	3.8
One-parent family	1.4	2.2	1.3	1.6	11.4	6.7	3.6	8.5	4.3
Complex household	4.4	6.1	4.6	4.9	3.5	6.0	7.5	5.0	5.0
Other	1.2	2.4	11.3	3.2	0.7	4.6	25.3	7.4	4.9
All (%)	100.0	100.0	100.0	100.0	100.0	100.0	100.0	100.0	100.0
All (N)	1,518	833	460	2,811	995	417	438	1,850	4,661

Source: ONS Longitudinal Study

and for women the percentages decline more sharply with age (43.8 per cent of women aged 26–34, 10.0 per cent of those aged 35–44, and 0 per cent for those aged 45–54). This difference is partly due to gender differences in the ages of partners (men are commonly older than the women with whom they live) and the fact that older women are less likely to have children young enough to be 'dependent'. Whereas none of the women living alone aged 45–54 in 1991 moved to 'couple with dependent children' households, in the younger age bands women are more likely than men to become lone parents.

The proportion of women moving from living alone to couple arrangements where there are no dependent children increases for women over the age of 35. The younger women are, like the younger men, moving from living alone to marrying/cohabiting prior to having children. The older women are most likely moving into households with men who had spent some time living alone if they left an earlier relationship.

The movements from different household arrangements to living alone and vice versa indicates a complex patterning of living alone across the life course of men and women. For both sexes there is a small group of people who live alone over long periods, whether through choice or from necessity, but for large numbers of people living alone is a transitional phase before or after cohabitation or marriage. This happens at different stages in the lives of women and men. Men are more likely to live alone earlier, after leaving marriage or cohabitation, whereas women are more likely to live alone later in life, after an interregnum of being a lone parent or due to widowhood.

Conclusion

This chapter provides an overview of the transitions to and from living alone. It also indicates the methodological possibilities and limitations of using longitudinally linked Census data to follow movements in and out of living alone. While living alone is only one of several household formations, it is the one which is growing fastest and has consequent implications for our understanding of families and communities, as well as for resource allocation in social care and housing in particular.

That an increasing number of people were living alone was known prior to this research. However, through using longitudinal data from the last 30 years, we have been able to show the patterning and increasing prevalence of living alone over the life course for many people. The data presented here have limitations and can only provide us with decennial 'snapshots' of people's household living arrangements. However, it is important to remember that these are the *same* people and we are therefore following their household transitions across long periods of their lives. The analyses can tell us nothing about motivations for moves into or out of living alone, or indeed remaining in that state. Nevertheless, that we can chart these moves suggests both fruitful avenues for further investigation and a basis for further theorisation.

These findings help to contextualise some of the theoretical writings mentioned earlier. For example, notions of individualisation may be associated with less permanent household arrangements, but shifts to living alone appear to be a complex phenomenon and not all moves are lifestyle choices. For younger people, it seems likely that living alone prior to marriage or cohabitation is a lifestyle choice, but this is less the case for people in older age groups. For example, the move from 'nuclear family' type households to living alone is gendered, with women more likely to experience this at a later point than men. Men are more likely to live alone earlier in their lives after the break-up of marriage or cohabitation. For women, after such break-up, living alone is usually postponed until after their children leave home. In both cases there may be no specific decision to live alone, but rather this is the unintended consequence of the choosing of other household arrangements by former household members.

Living alone, amongst young people, is concentrated in urban areas and in professional classes. For young professionals, particularly those on the economic 'escalator' (Fielding 1992) living alone may be clearly chosen, but equally it is not a choice open to many other youngsters who have great difficulty in affording to rent alone or buy property. Therefore, the flip side to the choice of living alone, for young people, is the lack of opportunity for many to do so. Given suitable housing opportunities, would more young people choose to live alone than is the case at present?

These differences in the patterning of living alone have implications for economic independence, friendship, and support networks, which tend to be different for men and women. Social networks, levels of support, and contact will be shaped by gender in different ways at different points in the life course, but also through social class, child-rearing responsibilities, and access to suitable housing.

Our analyses necessitated a very clear definition of what constituted living alone, but this cannot reflect the diversity of individual circumstances amongst those who live alone. In particular there is an inevitable blurring of the boundaries between living alone and cohabitation. At least some people who spend a part of their lives sharing living arrangements would have reported themselves as living alone on the Census form and vice versa. More research is needed to explore the nature of the living arrangements of those enumerated as 'living alone' and their connections with others and the wider community.

These caveats indicate that although living alone is one of the most profound demographic characteristics of our era, there is much work to be done. The foregoing is a modest attempt using longitudinal data to provide descriptions of moves into and out of living alone in England and Wales that might serve as a useful basis for further sociological and policy-related research and analyses.

Notes

1 The school leaving age in 1971.
2 Women of 40 or older in 1981 would have reached retirement age by 2001.
3 A separate longitudinal study based on Scottish Census data was relaunched in 2006.
4 36–44 in 2001.
5 Strictly speaking these are 'LS members' living in households. As a proportion of total number of persons they would be less because all other household types contain more than one person.
6 In this case the additional adult is most likely to be the LS member now living alone.
7 36–44 in 2001.

References

Allan, G. and Crow, G. (2001) *Families, households and society*, Basingstoke: Palgrave.
Allan, G. and Jones, G. (eds) (2003) *Social relations and the life course*, Basingstoke: Palgrave.
Bauman, Z. (2003) *Liquid love*, Cambridge: Polity Press.
Bawin-Legros, B. (2001) 'Families in Europe: A private and political stake – intimacy and solidarity', *Current Sociology*, 49: 49–65.
Bawin-Legros, B. (2004) 'Intimacy and the new sentimental order', *Current Sociology*, 52: 241–50.
Beck, U. and Beck-Gernsheim, E. (1995) *The normal chaos of love*, Cambridge: Polity.
Beck, U. and Beck-Gernsheim, E. (2002) *Individualization: institutionalized individualism and its social and political consequences*, London: Sage.
Beck-Gernsheim, E. (2002) *Reinventing the family: in search of new lifestyles*, Cambridge: Polity.
Chandler, J., Williams, M., Maconachie, M., Collett, T. and Dodgeon, B. (2004) 'Living alone: its place in household formation and change', *Sociological Research On Line* 9(3): http://www.socresonline.org.uk/9/3/chandler.html
Collett, T., Williams, M., Maconachie, M., Chandler, J. and Dodgeon, B. (2006) 'Long termness with regards to sickness and disability: an example of the value of longitudinal data for testing reliability and validity', *International Journal of Social Research Methodology, Theory and Practice*, 9(3): 224–43.
Dale, A., Williams, M. and Dodgeon, B. (1996) *Housing deprivation and social change*, London: HMSO.
Fielding, A. (1992) 'Migration and social mobility: South East England as an escalator region', *Regional Studies*, 26(1): 1–15.
Giddens, A. (1992) *The transformation of intimacy*, Cambridge: Polity Press.
Giele, J. Z. and Elder, G. H. (eds) (1998) *Methods of life course research: qualitative and quantitative approaches*, Sage: London.
Gittins, D. (1985) *The family in question*, Basingstoke: Macmillan.
Goldscheider, F. and Waite, L. (1991) *New families, no families*, Berkeley: University of California.

Hattersley, L. and Creeser, R. (1995) *LS Series 7: Longitudinal Study 1971–1991. History, organisation and quality of data*, London: HMSO.

Hooper, A., Dunmore, K. and Hughes, M. (1998) 'The housing preferences of one-person households' in *Home alone*, vol. 1, London: The Housing Research Foundation.

Jamieson, L., Stewart, L., Anderson, M., Bechofer, F. and Mccrone, D. (2003) 'Single, 20-something and seeking?' in G. Allan and G. Jones (eds) *Social relations and the life course*, Basingstoke: Palgrave.

Kaufmann, J. C. (1994) 'One person households in Europe', *Population*, 49(4–5): 935–58.

Levin, I. (2004) 'Living apart together: a new family form', *Current Sociology*, 52: 223–40.

Office for National Statistics (2003) *Social trends 33*: http://www.statistics.gov.uk/socialtrends

Overton, E. and Ermisch, J. (1984) 'Minimal household units', *Population Trends* No 35, London: OPCS.

Roseneil, S. and Budgeon, S. (2004) 'Cultures of intimacy and care beyond "the family": personal life and social change in the early 21st century', *Current Sociology*, 52: 135–59.

Silva, E. and Smart, C. (eds) (1999) *The New Family?*, London: Sage.

Strode, M. (1998) 'Analysis of 1993/4 and 1994/5 survey of English housing: single person households – the future and present characteristics' in *Home alone*, Vol. 2, London: The Housing Research Foundation.

Ware, L., Maconachie, M., Williams, M., Chandler, J. and Dodgeon, B. (2007) 'Gender Life Course Transitions from The Nuclear Family in England and Wales 1981–2001', *Sociological Research Online* 12(4): http://www.socresonline.org.uk/12/4/6.html

Williams, M. and Dale, A. (1991) 'Measuring housing deprivation using the OPCS Longitudinal Study', *LS Working Paper 72*, London: SSRU.

Williams, M. (2003) 'The problem of representation: realism and operationalism in survey research', *Sociological Research On Line* 8(1): http://www.socresonline.org.uk/8/1/williams.html

Acknowledgements

This article draws on research funded by the ESRC (RES-000–22–1413) under the Small Grants Scheme. The authors gratefully acknowledge the ONS for access to the Longitudinal Study.

Chapter 12

From educational priority areas to area-based interventions

Community, neighbourhood, and preschool[1]

Teresa Smith

Introduction

This chapter reviews the transformation of 'community' into 'area-based initiatives' over the last 50 years using the lens of the preschool policy developments of the Educational Priority Area Projects in the 1960s and the National Childcare Strategy of the 1990s as examples. The intention of this chapter is to review the definition and use of 'community' over the last 40 years as both the locus of the problem and the target for intervention. It focuses on two questions. First, what do we mean by 'community' and why is the idea so stubbornly persistent? Is it a myth, or a trick of political 'aerosol' (as Benington suggested with 'community school' or 'community policing', and others have suggested for 'community care'[2]), or does it have any substance? Second, does 'geographical community' continue to have importance as the locus for intervention, or has it been replaced by 'virtual community' (Macdonald and Grieco 2007)? Are neighbourhoods targeted because of the evidence on 'community as context' for people's life chances and life trajectories? Does where people live or work affect their educational outcomes, health, or earning potential, for example (Brooks-Gunn *et al.* 1997)? Is the neighbourhood the target because aspects of disadvantage are spatially distributed (a cost-effective strategy for reaching the largest number of disadvantaged families)?[3]

'Society is here/A true Community', wrote William Wordsworth in 1800 in the first volume of *The Recluse*, 'a genuine frame/Of many into one incorporate'. He was contrasting his close network of family and friends at home in Grasmere in the Lake District with urban life and 'the vast Metropolis ... /Where numbers overwhelm humanity/And neighbourhood serves rather to divide/Than to unite' (quoted in Sisman 2006). Wordsworth thereby reinforced the romantic notion of 'community' as a way of life that perhaps never entirely vanished. The idea of 'community' has a long history, as Raymond Williams[4] demonstrated in his *Keywords: a vocabulary of culture and society* (1976). Despite – or perhaps because of – its 'warm fuzziness', there have been many attempts at abolition, notably by Margaret

Stacey in the 1960s.[5] Stacey argued it was sociologically unnecessary as there was nothing about the term 'community' which could not be replaced by 'social relations' on the one hand, and 'locality' on the other. Nevertheless, she remained clear that the study of 'social relations in a locality' is important, perhaps equivalent to social networks or even social capital, in neighbourhoods. Others have been more sceptical about the concept the term is supposed to describe. Margaret Thatcher, for example, famously rubbished any notion of a collectivity beyond the individual and the family: 'There's no such thing as society. There are individual men and women, and there are families' (Thatcher, 1987: 8–10).

Yet 'community' has a stubborn persistence, both as a theoretical notion and in policy and politics. In social services, the Seebohm Report's (1968) vision of 'welfare through community', 'a community-oriented family service', and networks of 'reciprocal social relationships' as the basis for mutual aid was submerged in the introduction of local authorities' new social services departments in 1972. However, it re-emerged with the Barclay Report's (1982) support for decentralisation in the sense of locating services in the neighbourhood – 'going local' with small-scale, local 'patch' schemes (Hadley and McGrath 1980, 1984; Bayley et al. 1989; Smith 1989). These did not last as a local authority model, but 'community' and a community development approach to the provision of welfare has persisted alongside more individualised methods (Mayo 1994; Cannan and Warren 1997; Henderson 1995). This approach has re-appeared in Sure Start and the current development of Children's Centres, which are intended to be locally based, meeting the needs of their neighbourhoods. In local government in the 1980s, local authorities' moves to decentralise and democratise local services, labelled 'municipal socialism' (Boddy and Fudge 1984; Hoggett and Hambleton 1987; Seabrook 1984), in opposition to central government during Thatcher's heyday, prefigured programmes in the 1990s such as the New Deal for Communities and the 'compact' between local authorities and the voluntary and private sectors. More recently, 'community' has been captured by the Third Way (Etzioni 1997; Rose 2000), refashioned by the communitarians into 'social capital' (Frazer 1999; Schuller et al. 2000), utilised by New Labour as the basis for 'area-based initiatives' or neighbourhood targeting (Nash 2002, Nash with Christie 2002), and given a spatial measurement in the Index of Multiple Deprivation (DETR 2000, Noble et al. 2004).

We start with a brief sketch of the two time points. In the recent history of early years education and childcare in the UK there have been two periods of immense interest which are evident in a flurry of research activity and programme development. Both periods were stimulated by new thinking about the possibilities of boosting children's development, and intense debate about the relative weight of education and the environment, nature, and nurture. The first of these periods was the 1960s – a time in the USA when sociologists and psychologists were exploring how far the educational environment could influence children's cognitive development (Hunt 1961; Bloom 1964). The American War on Poverty saw the establishment of Head Start, a national programme for three- and four-year-old disadvantaged children that continues today. In the UK, the Plowden Report (CACE 1967) gave rise to the Educational Priority Areas Project (EPA). The EPA was established to address the educational underachievement of children from disadvantaged backgrounds (Halsey 1972; Smith *et al.* 2007a). The second period was the 1990s, when breakthroughs in the field of brain development demonstrated the importance of early experience in influencing the actual growth and development of neural pathways (e.g. Shonkoff and Phillips 2000). In the US, this was a factor in the introduction of Early Head Start to extend the Head Start intervention downwards and provide for children from pre-birth to school. In the UK, a number of area-based initiatives for young children and their families were launched under the wing of the 1998 National Childcare Strategy, including Sure Start and Neighbourhood Nurseries (now in the process of being 'rolled out' as mainstream services in Children's Centres). Thus key periods for early years in the UK were paralleled or preceded by developments in the USA, with interventions across the Atlantic generating interest and providing model programmes and important research evidence for UK counterparts.

Underlying and uniting these area-based early childhood initiatives in the US and the UK is the notion of 'community' as both the locus of the 'problem' and also the target for intervention. The driver for development of preschool services or early childhood interventions in the UK has primarily been child poverty and inequalities in life chances, in contrast to European states where there is more concern with demography and gender equity (Lewis and Campbell 2007). A long history in the UK of inequalities in educational outcomes has fuelled concern about inequalities in educational access and aspirations that all children should have 'equality of educational opportunity'. More recent concern to combat increasing levels of child poverty and inequality, particularly marked in the UK, is driving policy to enable more families with young children to enter employment through both supply-side and demand-side policies (i.e. with the help of publicly funded childcare and family support programmes, as well as tax credits and childcare credits for low income families in low-paid work). Services have been targeted, therefore, primarily at disadvantaged families suffering from income poverty.

EPAs and the rediscovery of community in the 1960s

The Educational Priority Areas Projects provide the first illustration of 'community-based interventions'. Launched in 1968 following the Plowden Report *Children and their primary schools* and focusing on 'positive discrimination' to target socially disadvantaged areas through educational policies, this was an early example of government-level intervention of the type now labelled 'area-based initiatives'. EPA's focus was on schools in run-down areas which had 'grim buildings, high staff turnover' and dispirited teachers, and used positive discrimination as a tool 'to make schools in the most deprived areas as good as the best in the country' (Halsey 1972). The idea was elaborated by Michael Young (later Lord Young of Dartington), drawing on both the American War on Poverty, with its Head Start programme then being developed for young children and their parents, and the UK tradition of community studies and small-scale innovation, brought together in the work of the Institute of Community Studies in East London since its foundation in 1954 with research by sociologists such as Peter Townsend, Norman Dennis, and Peter Willmott, as well as Michael Young himself (Frankenberg 1966; Bell and Newby 1971).

The 'rediscovery of community' in the 1950s and 1960s was illustrated by (now classic) studies such as *Family and kinship in East London* by Michael Young and Peter Willmott and *The family life of old people* by Peter Townsend, both set in Bethnal Green in Tower Hamlets (1957), and *Coal is our life* by Norman Dennis and colleagues (1956), which describes the community strengths, close relationships, and geography of pit and village in the Yorkshire coalfield. These studies vividly demonstrate the overlap between locality and kinship, and, in the Dennis study, occupation. Sociologically speaking they are as much studies of 'kin' as they are studies of 'community', located in small, close-knit, densely populated neighbourhoods characterised by a high level of face-to-face interaction and also continuity over a long period of time, where people knew a very high proportion of their neighbours and a very high proportion were inter-related, sometimes in three- or even four-generation families. 'Community' is defined as 'locality', characterised by 'length of residence or localised kinship', and marked by 'kinship, friendship and community spirit' (Young and Willmott 1957: 116, 198). Typically, community studies of this period took working-class neighbourhoods as their focus, and the 'rediscovery of community' was paralleled by the 'rediscovery of poverty'.[6] Shared values and shared experience were evident and rooted often in conditions of great deprivation: poverty, ill-health, poor housing, based on shared economic conditions, and, sometimes, dependence on a single industry such as mining, fishing, ship-building, and steel-making. Some of the EPA action-research projects were located in such areas.

The central notion of community is that 'people have something in common' – territory or locality, shared interests, or the rather more elusive notion 'sense of community' or 'spirit of community' (Willmott 1986: 83ff). Willmott calls the first notion 'place community' and the second 'interest community'; the third is more difficult to capture, to do with social relationships and perceptions: 'how many people feel a sense of identity with the place and of solidarity with the other people' (op. cit.). Thus 'community' does not just mean the locality or localities where people live, work, or socialise – that is more properly termed 'neighbourhood'. Nor does it just mean shared interests – that could be satisfied by the 'virtual community' of the global internet, without any geographical roots at all. The more elusive key element is the 'sense of identity' and the norms which people may share with a place, group, or even an idea. It is this sense that carries what Willmott calls 'rhetorical or moral overtones' – the 'caring community' appealed to so often by politicians and policy makers in which families, friends, and neighbours look after the old and needy, or the village-like communities of an earlier century where children walked safely on their own to school and people left their front doors unlocked. It also carries an implication of collective action: a community carries a history and may provide a base for local organisation (Leonard 1975).

When the three strands of 'community' (that is, locality or neighbourhood; social relations or family or social networks; and community spirit, norms or sense of identity) are examined in more detail, it is clear in the classic studies of community that they overlap. In the Bethnal Green studies of the late 1950s two out of three people interviewed had their parents living within two or three miles (in Bethnal Green itself or the neighbouring boroughs of Poplar, Stepney, or Shoreditch) and, on average, married women saw their mothers four times a week. A week's diary kept by one woman of the people she saw on her morning shopping trips down the street listed 63 people in all, 'some seen many times and thirty-eight of them relatives of at least one other person out of the sixty-three' (Young and Willmott 1957: 107). People who talked about 'moving away' were referring to distances of five or ten minutes' walk. Here, people said, 'you knew everybody, grew up with everybody, everybody recognised you' (Young and Willmott 1957: 102). This is a vivid picture of an area with long residence, close-knit kin, and a strong sense of community identity and community spirit. It is 'an orderly community based on family and neighbourhood groupings' and 'a village in the middle of London' (Willmott and Young 1960: 7). Very similar feelings are portrayed in the study of perceptions of community carried out in Sheffield in 1967 (Hampton 1970: 110–1), in parallel with the Royal Commission on Local Government's *Community Attitudes Survey* (1969). Four fifths of the national sample declared attachment to a home area, and this is how the Sheffield respondents described it:

> this street only and only as far as each corner on either side of this house; down the hill to Queens Road and back again; I feel at home here ... by the park and the shopping centre; I just go over the road to the bus to go to work.

The notion of 'community' was central to the Educational Priority Area Projects. The major determinants of educational attainment, wrote Halsey, its national director, are 'not schoolmasters but social situations, not curriculum but motivation, not formal access to the school but support in the family and the community'; 'the Plowden analysis of low educational standards in EPAs points to causes outside the school in the neighbourhood structure of life' (Halsey 1972: 4, 5). EPAs were an attempt to refashion the relationship between education and society. The goal of education should be the creation of a just society and equal access for all, whether this could be achieved by greater equality of opportunity or access to education, or by greater equality of educational achievement. Despite Bernstein's sharp criticism that 'education cannot compensate for society', Halsey remains open-minded as to the reforming capacity of education, and 'optimistic ... about the primary school and pre-school as points of entry for action-research aimed at inducing changes in the relation between school and community' (Halsey, 1972: 8). This is essentially a community analysis of educational opportunities and achievements. EPA strategies to develop pre-schooling and the community school were attempts to alter the relationship between school, family, and community, as well as to introduce new ways of defining and organising the learning environment.

EPA set up four action-research projects in England: in Deptford in London, central Liverpool, Balsall Heath in Birmingham, and Denaby Main/Conisbrough in South Yorkshire (Halsey 1972; Midwinter 1972; Barnes 1975; Smith 1975) (there was also a fifth in Scotland, in Dundee). These were small-scale projects which ran for three years, designed originally to target the 2 per cent (and intended to increase to the 10 per cent) of the most disadvantaged areas of the country. Each project put forward a different analysis of 'community'. For example, Denaby Main/Conisbrough in the West Riding EPA was an almost wholly white working-class area; the population was geographically very stable and there was very significant employment in the local pits and related industries. This was a community with strong vertical roots. According to the EPA surveys of parents, around 65 per cent of the mothers of primary school age children had been brought up in the same area. The area of inner Liverpool identified as the Liverpool EPA had a relatively small proportion of recent immigrants, but it was judged to be among the most deprived urban areas in England (some 28 per cent of the children in primary schools were able to claim free school meals, the highest among the four English EPAs), but it was also an area with strong vertical roots (60 per cent of mothers were brought up in the same area). Both Deptford and Birmingham EPAs were marked by more recent mobility, with fewer parents claiming to be from the same area – particularly so in Birmingham, where almost a third of the residents had been born outside Great Britain. Thus the EPAs differed markedly in the stability or movement of the population, length of residence, and sense of identity with an area.

The West Riding EPA provides a more detailed example. As in Dennis's earlier study of a mining community, Denaby Main/Conisbrough stood out for its close identification with the mining industry. Tight-knit friendship and family networks were strong, and there was a clear highly localised identity. 'Here' was contrasted with 'not here, but across the street'; a daughter had left home and 'gone away' – to the next town, just over the railway crossing. One quarter of the parents surveyed had attended their child's current school; 45 per cent of the families had lived in the same house for 15 years or more; more than 60 per cent had many of their relatives living near by, and more than 80 per cent had many of their friends also living near by; 95 per cent of the children played with local children after school. Teachers also tended to live locally, with more than one in five living less than half a mile from the school where they taught. Most of this reads more like Bethnal Green than the Birmingham or Deptford EPAs. The question is what this meant for parents' expectations and understanding of education, and for children's educational potential and performance. On the whole, parents expected to leave 'teaching' (that is, 'learning useful things' and educating children 'so that they can get a good job') to the school; 'he learns nothing from me – he'll learn when he goes to school' was an attitude frequently expressed by parents; 50 per cent thought that their views on education were shared by other parents – more than in the other EPAs.

The EPA example shows that 'community' was seen not only as the target for intervention, but also as the locus of the problem. Parents thought education was important and wanted to do the best for their children. However, both teachers' and parents' expectations were low, and there seemed to be little understanding of the importance of the social situations, motivation, and support in the family and the community. As Halsey set out, expectations and attitudes are rooted in the particular community, and educational programmes have to take that into account.

We should remember that data of the kind now routinely available to measure disadvantage at the local level through the Index of Multiple Deprivation was largely restricted to the census in the 1950s and 1960s. The EPA areas and schools for study were selected largely on professional judgement; the one attempt at systematic measurement of deprivation as a basis for selection was carried out by the Inner London Education Authority (see Halsey 1972; Smith *et al.* 2007a; Payne 1974). The more detailed descriptions of geography and attitudes, areas and families, parents and teachers, and schools and their neighbourhoods in Townsend's and Young and Willmott's studies of Bethnal Green, Hampton's study in Sheffield, and the studies of the Yorkshire coalfield carried out by Dennis and his colleagues, as well as the EPA studies, required surveys carried out specially for the research. What has changed some 50 years later is the richness of the routinely available administrative data to supplement the census at both national and local level.

We can now see, with hindsight, that the neighbourhoods that provided the focus and location for the EPAs at the end of the 1960s were very diverse and already changing. In Denaby Main/Conisbrough, the first of the national strikes in the mining industry that contributed to its decline and collapse under the Thatcher governments took place during the EPA period. This provided a sharp commentary on the relationship between home and school, which is as relevant now as it was then. Schools closed because they depended on coal; parents said they could not think about their children's learning when they did not know where the next meal was coming from. Education and the economy are intertwined.

Revisiting 'community' in the 1990s

Nearly 50 years later, can we say that such geographical communities still exist? The working-class neighbourhoods bound together by kinship, common occupation, and adversity depicted by Young and Willmott and others have declined or fragmented. This was already happening in the 1950s with the migration of young Bethnal Green families to the new London County Council housing estates such as 'Greenleigh' out in Essex (Young and Willmott 1957). Twenty years on, fragmentation seemed to be gathering pace. Just about a third of the sample in the 1977 Lambeth Inner Area Study felt they belonged to a 'local neighbourhood' (Shankland et al. 1977: 39). Interviews carried out at the end of the 1970s with people and community groups in four inner London boroughs (Knight and Hayes 1981: 30) revealed high levels of social isolation and social disintegration: 'I don't like anything about this area. I'm just living here because I have to live here, I have no alternative. If I had, I wouldn't be here.' But community spirit may be more a matter of growth than planning. As Hampton pointed out in the 1967 Sheffield study, over the years residents of the 'new housing estates' may develop just as strong community identity as older more traditional neighbourhoods.

Two studies of 'community' published in the new millennium, both deliberate 'revisits' of the earlier Bethnal Green research, reveal some of the changes over the last 50 years and also demonstrate differences not only over time but also between areas. Mumford and Power studied two neighbourhoods of Hackney and Newham through interviews with 100 families and portrayed them in *East Enders: family and community in East London* (2003) (see also Lupton and Power 2002; Richardson and Mumford 2002). Dench, Gavron, and Michael Young[7] at the Institute of Community Studies published *The new East End: kinship, race and conflict* (2006). It was originally planned as a repeat of the 1953 survey and commissioned in 1992 with the same questions on family life and neighbourhood, but was transformed over the next ten years into a study of ethnic diversity and conflict. What do these studies tell us about the decline and fragmentation of 'community' or its continuity and strength?

Mumford and Power set out to explore why neighbourhoods 'matter' – 'the impact of poor neighbourhood conditions on family life' – and the overlap between neighbourhood and community. Their language of community is similar to the older study: 'relating "community" to "neighbourhood" fuses social networks with geography, suggesting the existence of shared interests and/or identity in shared space'. Their conclusions are that 'community spirit' is still perceived as important (rated as such by more than four-fifths of their sample). Thirty per cent spoke of it as friendship enhancing the quality of life, to do with tolerance and mixing, 25 per cent as informal help and bringing people together. Four in ten people felt part of the community because they attended church or other groups, or helped with children's activities or at school, or because they worked locally. 'Community' meant 'helping neighbours, feeling safe, bringing people together, making people responsible, joining in, making things work, cooperating, overcoming barriers, seeing familiar friendly faces' (Mumford and Power 2003: 55). This was particularly important for mothers with young children. But there are two crucial differences from the earlier Bethnal Green: family structure and ethnic diversity. In Mumford and Power's study, kinship networks received little attention, and half the study respondents were lone mothers, while the areas in Hackney and Newham have become much more ethnically mixed. This has led to competition particularly for housing and education. Despite these changes, however, Mumford and Power's study suggests that 'community', at least for groups such as young mothers, remains strong as social networks with friends and neighbours even in the absence of family, and for many people it transcends ethnic differences.

Dench, Gavron, and Young's study tells a rather different story. It documents the segmentation of the East End, following immigration, economic decline, and regeneration over the last 30 years, into separate communities of older white families and younger Bangladeshi families. While the large extended families and kinship networks typical of the earlier Bethnal Green study had largely vanished from the white community (with smaller families, more lone parents, and housing shortages which meant young people moving away), such family networks were now more typical of the Bangladeshi community. Conflict was based on competition for work, but more importantly, according to this study as in that by Mumford and Power, conflict was also based on competition for access to resources from the state, such as housing and education. Educational achievement and expectations were different too. Bangladeshis outperformed the English, Scottish, and Welsh (ESW) group and also the Tower Hamlet average: local authority figures for 2002 show that 46 per cent of Bangladeshi students achieved five GCSE A+ to C grades compared with 30 per cent of the ESW group and 42 per cent of Tower Hamlets students overall. Teachers valued Bangladeshi parents for the discipline and educational aspirations they instilled in their children, particularly the girls, who 'value education … as a way of improving their life chances. They see that quite early on. And they work very, very hard' (Dench et al. 2006: 141, 142).

These two studies demonstrate some of the changes in 'community' and social cohesion over the last 50 years, but also the differences within and between small areas within a large and multi-cultural city such as London. 'Community' of a kind, for some groups, remains strong in both areas, though it is clearly bound up with access to resources. Young mothers in Mumford and Power's study may not have to compete for the local playgroup or the coffee morning, but when it comes to housing or school places, both studies suggest it is a different matter. This may give a new angle to the emphasis in earlier studies that 'community' was born out of adversity, war, harsh material circumstances, or dangerous occupations (Willmott 1986: 91, 96). In the later studies the struggle may be for access to the resources of the welfare state (e.g. education and social housing). This is a fresh angle on the economic base of 'community'.

We should note, however, that these two studies have rather different conceptions of community and use rather different methods. While both studies document their multi-ethnic neighbourhoods, that by Dench and colleagues provides a denser historical analysis of the changes over the last 50 years, particularly in family structure and social networks in both white and minority ethnic communities. Mumford and Power's work is a small study of 100 families, using opportunistic sampling ('snowballing') to recruit families through doctors' surgeries and local primary schools, against a backdrop of interviews with schools, police, community organisations, churches, and health workers, and observations of meetings (Mumford and Power 2003: Figure 2.3). It is a qualitative study, deliberately told through 'what people have to say for themselves', their 'feelings and reactions to life in their neighbourhoods', 'rather than the wider academic debates of a more theoretical nature about regeneration and community relations' (Mumford and Power 2003: 3). The study by Dench and colleagues is a far larger and more rigorous study, with data on about 8,000 people, based on interviews with 799 households drawn from a large random sample picked from the electoral register, followed up by more intensive interviews with 51 respondents, as well as interviews with local teachers, youth workers, and council officials (Dench et al. 2006: 235ff). While this study also uses interviews, they illustrate the argument rather than create the argument itself.

Community, social capital, ABIs, and New Labour

The election of the New Labour government in 1997 marked a swing of the policy pendulum back to 'community' as the focus for intervention. 'Area-based initiatives' (rapidly shortened to ABIs) were seen as the answer to the 'geography of disadvantage' described in the reports by the newly established Social Exclusion Unit (1998). The poor neighbourhoods described had more than their share of unemployment, poor housing, high levels of lone parent households, children growing up in families on benefit, ethnic minorities, poor literacy, school leavers with low grades, and poorly performing schools. Residents complained of crime, vandalism, litter, pollution, poor shops and public transport, lack of community spirit, and unsupervised youngsters on the streets. A national strategy to 'turn around poor neighbourhoods' was announced. The strategy already included the New Deal for Communities and Education/Health/Employment Action Zones. Sure Start was intended to bring together health, education, and welfare for young children and their families in the most disadvantaged neighbourhoods of the country.

The policy rationale for this revived focus on the 'geography of disadvantage' relies heavily on three things. First, it draws on the increasingly detailed data now available at national level (in contrast to the 1960s) which has focused attention on the inequalities between the most and least advantaged areas in the country, trends over time, and the stubborn persistence of poverty and deprivation both at a regional level and in small pockets in the wealthiest neighbourhoods (Noble and Smith 1996). The 'rediscovery of community' by the Labour government post-1997 mirrors the 'rediscovery of community' in the 1950s and 1960s (although there seems little evidence of awareness by politicians of such precedents). Second, it draws explicitly on research, particularly on young children's development, demonstrating the gap in life chances between children growing up in poverty and those growing up in well-off families in well-off neighbourhoods (e.g. Bradshaw and Mayhew 2005; Sylva et al. 2004). Third, it builds on assumptions about 'community', or lack of it, and the importance of 'capacity building' and 'social capital' for building up individual skills and strong self-sufficient neighbourhoods (e.g. SEU 1998: 57; Taylor 1995).

The detailed socio-demographic data not available in the 1960s but now widely available is drawn from the Index of Multiple Deprivation (DETR 2000; Noble et al. 2004), which combines indicators on a number of domains (including income, employment, health, education, housing and services, environment, and crime) to measure deprivation at a small area level. Each 'domain' combines a number of 'indicators'. The 2004 'Income Deprivation Domain', for example, includes adult and children in households receiving Income Support (IS), Income Based Job Seekers Allowance JSA(IB), Working Families Tax Credit (WFTC; now Working Tax Credit [WTC]), Disabled Persons' Tax Credit (DPTC), and asylum seekers. Data sources include the Department for Work and Pensions (DWP), Inland Revenue, the Home Office, and the National Asylum Support Service (NASS). The Income Deprivation Affecting Children (IDAC) Index is a subset of the Income Deprivation Domain and includes the proportion of children under 16 in families receiving IS or JSA (IB) or WFTC/ DPTC, living below 60 per cent of median income (Noble et al. 2004: 18–9).

The advantages of this type of routinely collected administrative data are that it is consistent and robust, and allows comparison between different types of 'neighbourhoods' and of change and continuity in neighbourhoods over time. All data is postcoded, and can be aggregated 'up' or 'down' into geographical units of whatever size is required. (In ID 2004, Super Output Areas [SOAs] with a population of about 1,500 people replaced wards as the smallest geographical unit for which data is routinely made available.) IMD data allows the government to target public funds across the country,[8] and allows local authorities to target areas of deprivation. 'Postcode data', through IDAC, for example, allows us to document the inequitable distribution of children's life chances with much greater detail and precision than could be done by the EPA studies of the 1960s. But administrative data does not include the information on attitudes or social networks needed to analyse 'community'. For this, we continue to rely on surveys, as in the 1960s.

The capture of 'community' by the communitarians and the Third Way in the guise of 'capacity building' and 'social capital', which has emerged in the 1990s as the basis for area-based policies, may just be a currently fashionable relabelling, but it carries different 'baggage'[9] (for another perspective see Chapter 5 this volume). As first formulated by Coleman (1988), Bourdieu (1986) and Putnam (2000) (see also Schuller *et al.* 2000), social capital is defined in parallel to, but distinct from, economic capital on the one hand and human capital on the other. For some, it is an individual attribute (people's individual contacts help them get jobs). For others, social capital belongs to groups or communities (e.g. the density of formal and informal groups). Social capital thus invites us to focus on social relations and the purposes for which people engage in social networks: to improve education; to get a job; or to create a clean water supply. The 'networks, norms and social trust' that facilitate co-ordination and collaboration for mutual benefit may or may not have a geographical overlap. The justification of interest in social capital is spelt out in terms very similar to the justification of interest in community: high levels of social capital have been found to be correlated with good health, lower crime rates, higher educational achievement, strong economic performance, and so on. Thus 'social capital', like 'community', may be understood as both the context for such desirable outcomes and also as the focus for intervention in order to achieve such outcomes.

Putnam's conclusions on the decline of social capital and the rise of individualism in the USA are supported by more recent analysis (McPherson *et al.* discussed in Macdonald and Grieco 2007) and have been widely quoted. But any claim for universal applicability has been questioned. Analysis of the British Social Attitudes surveys, for example, suggests Britain still has a more robust civil society (Johnston and Jowell 2001; Haezewindt 2003). However, together with the increasing interest in the UK in evidence-based policy and revived concern with community and neighbourhood, the notion of social capital has focused attention on existing data sources available to measure key dimensions such as reciprocity and trust, citizenship and civic participation, neighbourliness, social networks and support, volunteering, and social participation, as well as people's views about living in an area. The UK General Household Survey (GHS) provides a detailed example.

GHS 2000 included a component on 'social capital' (Coulthard *et al.* 2002). Key findings from the 2000 survey showed that the longer people had lived in an area, the stronger their neighbourliness and social networks, but the more likely they were to be critical of local services and to report high levels of local problems. But groups varied by class and ethnicity. Most importantly for our analysis of disadvantaged neighbourhoods, levels of social capital tended overall to decrease as levels of disadvantage rose. People living in the 10 per cent most disadvantaged neighbourhoods were less likely to show or feel civic engagement, or to trust people in the neighbourhood, and were more likely to be victims of crime and to rate their neighbourhoods poor on facilities and high on problems. But generalisations mask significant differences. For example, people in the least deprived neighbourhoods were more likely to have a generalised sense of 'trusting strangers' – almost three-quarters said they would trust most or many people in the neighbourhood – while those living in the most deprived neighbourhoods were more likely to have a specific sense of trust – nearly half said they would trust 'a few' people. Collective action and a sense of power was not monopolised by the well-off: more than half of those living in the most disadvantaged neighbourhoods thought that local people could influence decisions that affected the neighbourhood, and more than a quarter said they had taken action to solve local problems. The biggest exception to the general trends in social capital concerned the localised nature of social networks. People living in the most disadvantaged neighbourhoods were far more likely to speak to their neighbours every day (33 per cent compared to 19 per cent in the least deprived neighbourhoods), to have close relatives living nearby, to see and telephone them every day, and also to see and telephone friends. Curiously, however, these social networks seemed less likely to provide social support in times of illness or financial difficulty, for example.

To some extent, these findings reassuringly demonstrate the continuing strength of 'community' in Britain, including locality, strong social networks, and some aspects of civic engagement. But they also suggest rather more nuanced distinctions between more disadvantaged and more affluent neighbourhoods – for example, in the meaning of 'social trust'. Other studies are more cautious. Trends in involvement reported in the BSA surveys, such as membership or volunteering, and in social trust, suggest two things. First, although there is little evidence of the decline in organisational membership found by Putnam in the USA (apart from religious affiliation and trade unions), there does seem to have been a decline in social trust over the last 40 years. Second, there is a familiar pattern of greater involvement by the better-off. As Johnston and Jowell demonstrate, the 'well-heeled' are more likely not only to be 'joiners' (involved in organisations such as

Neighbourhood Watch schemes, Parent–Teacher Associations, school governing bodies, etc.), but also to have higher levels of social trust. If social capital is patterned along class lines, it may serve to reinforce social divisions rather than create social cohesion (see Hall in Putnam 2002). This reminds us of Putnam's distinction between 'bonding' and 'bridging' capital, and his more recent work on the social distribution of social capital and the importance of ethnicity in how social capital operates differently in different communities (Putnam 2002). The study of the East End by Dench and his colleagues distinguishes between the more fragmented traditional white working class and the more educationally successful Bangladeshis. Social capital in the sense of social networks, community norms, and aspirations may be strong in both communities but with different outcomes.

'Community', ABIs, and Labour's National Childcare Strategy: Sure Start and the Neighbourhood Nursery Initiative (NNI)

Ten years of the Labour government's National Childcare Strategy gives us a lens through which to view the most recent transformation of 'community'. Sure Start, later renamed Sure Start Local Programmes (SSLPs), and the Neighbourhood Nursery Initiative (NNI) have both been claimed as examples of 'community-based interventions' and 'area-based initiatives', targeting disadvantaged neighbourhoods[10] (like the EPAs of the 1960s). How was 'community' defined in Sure Start and NNI, and what was the rationale for intervention?

Both programmes have been well targeted in the most disadvantaged neighbourhoods of the country. Sure Start areas (524 of them by the end of the programme) were significantly more deprived than the area average for England, as characterised by lower income, more child poverty, more crime, lower educational achievement, higher birth rates, more lone-parent families and teenage parents, and poorer child and adult health. Over time there has been significant change in Sure Start areas with more childcare, fewer families reliant on benefits, better educational results, and fewer children hospitalised for severe injury (Barnes *et al.* 2003, 2007), although the data do not allow us to make a causal claim. This change is set against a backdrop of country-wide improvement over the period in numbers of low-income families with preschool children dependent on out-of-work means-tested benefits (Sigala and Smith 2007). NNI aimed to increase childcare in disadvantaged areas to help low-income parents, particularly mothers, back into work and so reduce child poverty. Three-quarters of the 1,400 neighbourhood nurseries were located in the 30 per cent most disadvantaged neighbourhoods, and NNI has reached some of the most disadvantaged groups (low income families, lone parents, ethnic minority families, and parents with low qualifications in particular) (Smith *et al.* 2007b). The rationale for both programmes was thus clearly a cost-effective strategy to reach large numbers of highly disadvantaged families. In the case of Sure Start the strategy was to develop a more integrated approach to providing health, education, and welfare services for young children and their families, while in the case of NNI the strategy was to provide childcare in such areas. Both programmes have been largely successful in their targeting, although longer-term impact for children and parents remains to be seen.

'Community' is more difficult to define or locate in either programme. Areas were selected and defined in both on the basis of IMD data which, as we have seen, does not include 'social capital'-type information, and there was no attempt to collect such data systematically.[11] 'Community' has been highly contentious in Sure Start. On the one hand, some critics point to the distortion of the original programme by the shift away from earlier objectives of 'community development/parental control' (Glass 2006). On the other hand, there are problems for area-based interventions such as Sure Start in adopting a very open-ended 'community development' approach without a clear 'programme' (Rutter 2006).

However, in two senses it may be argued that these initiatives were indeed intended to be about 'community'. First, both were explicitly area-based rather than individually based programmes: their services were open to all families with children in the right age group living in the neighbourhood. Second, both were sensitive, in different ways, to community context and community variation – that people defined their needs differently and made different use of services in different types of area, and that services should be 'tailor-made' to the local area. The NNI findings (Smith *et al.* 2007c) show examples of nurseries providing part-time care, charging sessional fees to meet the needs of particular labour markets, or offering 'tasters' in some minority ethnic communities to draw in women with young children who were not expected to go out to work. Sure Start was explicitly described as a 'community development approach' based on partnership between local people and professionals. Early findings (NESS 2005a, 2005b) suggest the style and context of different projects was important, with *empowerment* (local users and community groups involved in service planning, and staff and users working as a 'learning community') associated with less negative parenting at nine months, and good *identification of users* (strategies to reach potential users, multi-agency working such as information sharing, and support for children with special needs) associated with improved child outcomes at three years. But community-based strategies for intervention need to be more systematically developed and understood.[12]

Conclusion

There are a number of assumptions underpinning area-based or community-based approaches that have to be disentangled: the nature of 'community' itself and the relationship between 'individual' and 'community' or 'neighbourhood' levels of analysis and intervention, for example. When we compare the 1960s and the late 1990s, it is clear there has to be a coherent theoretical model about how 'community' operates, the economic, social, and normative dimensions that are important, and the processes and the structures (e.g. family and peer groups) that mediate how children learn and behave (Brooks-Gunn et al. 1997; Lupton and Power 2002; Richardson and Mumford 2002). (For EPA, Halsey set out well-articulated models of the relationship between education and society, as well as between home, community, and educational achievement. In the 1990s, programmes such as Sure Start are more complex, and theoretical models are less well spelt out. 'Parental involvement' and 'empowerment' are 'buzz words' in Sure Start, for example, but so far there has been little work published on the theoretical complexities of these concepts.) This chapter has argued that 'neighbourhood' and 'community' operate not only as convenient geographical shorthand for policy interventions (because of local concentrations of disadvantaged families and young children), but also as theoretical concepts, which may drive or mediate processes (because of the effects of different contexts). We have seen the importance of distinguishing these two meanings of 'neighbourhood as locality', and 'neighbourhood effects' or 'neighbourhood as context'.

The relationship between 'individual' and 'community' or 'neighbourhood' levels of analysis and intervention remains complex. The ecological fallacy is still alive and kicking[13], although it should be well understood that to define areas as disadvantaged does not mean everyone living in such areas is disadvantaged, and there will be disadvantaged people living outside such areas. What do we mean by 'community-level programmes' or 'community-based analysis'? Halsey argued that the EPA programmes were 'natural experiments' which combined the individual child, the school, and the neighbourhood as distinct 'units' of analysis.

> The area approach is based on recognising the complex forces in school and community which determine the meaning and effectiveness of educational experience including attainment. It also recognises that schooling is more than the transmission and competitive testing of academic skills.
>
> (Halsey 1972: 43ff)

EPA did, however, also include forms of randomisation as well as matched research designs (children were randomly allocated to some treatments, and the nationally adopted preschool programme was randomly allocated to nurseries), and its testing programmes of children, surveys of parents and teachers, and comparative data on communities were rigorous in collection and analysis. Randomised controlled trials (RCTs) are now well known within community level programmes. There are examples in both Early Head Start in the USA and Sure Start in the UK (Love *et al.* 2005; Hutchings *et al.* 2007). In north and mid-Wales, for example, where eleven Sure Start projects now use the Webster-Stratton Incredible Years parenting programme, 153 families agreeing to take part were randomly allocated; in Early Head Start, 3,000 families across 17 sites took part.

Two conclusions can be drawn from this overview. The first conclusion is that there is still evidence for both 'geographical community' and 'communities of interest' existing in the new millennium, even if it is fragmented and conflicted (e.g. compare Bethnal Green in the 1960s and the 1990s). There are also more powerful methods of measurement of both the physical and the 'social capital' components of community through routinely collected administrative and survey data, and also of 'intervention outcomes' through randomised controlled trials using techniques which are sensitive to area variations. The second conclusion is that 'community' still provides an important focus for interventions, although we need to understand community norms and expectations more clearly. The assumptions underlying area-based initiatives are that disadvantage is concentrated, and some services, such as schools and health services, are area-based. Services need to be tailored for (and, perhaps, controlled by) local areas, as was grasped by the EPA projects in the 1960s and 'patch-based' local authorities in the 1980s, and has been built in to Sure Start and Children's Centres. Perhaps, as demonstrated by the Bangladeshis in Tower Hamlets, it is the communities that are already more cohesive, where community and family objectives chime with the objectives of public services such as schools, which offer the most fertile ground for successful outcomes. The challenge is how to intervene where 'community' is fragmented, groups are in competition, and objectives are potentially in conflict.

Notes

1 I am grateful to Emily Tanner for her collaboration on an earlier version of this chapter given as a paper to the Social Policy Association's conference 27-29 June 2005.

2 Abrams (1978), in his seminal article on 'community care', suggests the fault is confusion rather than rhetoric, and distinguishes between services 'located in the community' (as in 'outreach' or 'domiciliary' services provided by professionals placed 'in the community'), services 'provided by the community' (as in meals-on-wheels provided by local people), and small-scale residential centres provided in a small, local, friendly, and informal format (the deliberately constructed 'caring community').

3 Although there will always be disadvantaged individuals outside the most disadvantaged areas: for example, only 54 per cent of poor children lived in the 20 per cent most deprived wards according to the Index of Multiple Deprivation 2000 (see Work and Pensions Select Committee 2003, para.43).

4 Williams summed up 'community' as 'the warmly persuasive word to describe an existing set of relationships, or the warmly persuasive word to describe an alternative set of relationships. What is most important, perhaps, is that unlike all other terms of social organisation (state, nation, society, etc.) it seems never to be used unfavourably, and never to be given any positive opposing or distinguishing term.'

5 Stacey, M. (1969) endorsed Hillery's refusal to use the word 'community' because it 'embraces a motley assortment of concepts and qualitatively different phenomena'. Hillery (1963) was famous for his 94 definitions of 'community'.

6 Popular imagination and indignation was caught by the 'rediscovery of poverty' portrayed by Abel-Smith and Townsend (1965) and Townsend and Wedderburn (1965). Moorhouse (1964) echoed Harrington's study (1962), which was credited with helping to spark America's War on Poverty. Poverty studies in the style we might call 'the documentary novel' (rather than the literary study of 'community in the novel' - see, for example, Killham 1977) continued throughout the 1970s and 1980s - Coates and Silburn's survey of St Ann's in Nottingham (1970); Harrison's documentary on Hackney (1983) and Parker's interviews on a South London housing estate (1983); and Campbell (1984) harking back to George Orwell's 1937 account of poverty in the Depression, *The Road to Wigan Pier.*

7 Michael Young died in 2002. The Institute of Community Studies has been renamed The Young Foundation.

8 Latest estimates suggest between 1 and 2 per cent of public expenditure is distributed via the IMD.

9 What we mean by 'baggage' is neatly encapsulated in Jules Feiffer's 1965 cartoon about deprivation (reproduced in Smith and Noble 1995: 28): the description changes but the problem remains the same.

10 Both programmes have now been 'rolled up' into Sure Start Children's Centres.

11 Although Barnes *et al.* (2003, 2007) analyse large amounts of administrative data to establish a typology of different types of disadvantaged areas.

12 See Craig *et al.* (2007) for a critical analysis of Sure Start's understanding of black and ethnic minority communities. See also Belsky *et al.* (2007).

13 See note 3. The ecological fallacy refers to the assumption that individual level characteristics can be inferred from area level characteristics and vice versa.

References

Abel-Smith, B. and Townsend, P. (1965) *The poor and the poorest: a new analysis of the Ministry of Labour's Family Expenditure Surveys of 1953–54 and 1960,* London: Bell.

Abrams, P. (1978) 'Community care: some research problems and priorities', in Barnes, J. and Connolly, N. (eds) *Social Care Research,* London: PSI/Bedford Square Press.

Barclay Report (1982) *Social workers: their roles and tasks,* London: Bedford Square Press.

Barnes, J. (1975) *Educational priority: volume 3: curriculum innovation in London's EPAs,* London: HMSO.

Barnes, J., Broomfield, K., Frost, M., Harper, G., McLeod, A., Knowles, J. and Leyland, A. (2003) *Characteristics of Sure Start local programme areas: Rounds 1 to 4*, London: Department for Education and Skills.

Barnes, J., Cheng, H., Howden, B., Frost, M., Harper, G., Lattin-Rawstrone, R., Sack, C. and the NESS team (2007) *Changes in the characteristics of SSLP areas between 2000/01 and 2004/05*, Research report NESS/2007/FR/021, London: Department for Education and Skills.

Bayley, M., Seyd, R. and Tennant, A. (1989) *Local health and welfare: is partnership possible? – a study of the Dinnington Project*, Aldershot: Gower.

Bell, C. and Newby, H. (1971) *Community studies: an introduction to the sociology of the local community*, London: Allen and Unwin.

Belsky, J., Bornes, J. and Melhuish, E. (eds) (2007) *The National Evaluation of Sure Start: does area-based early intervention work?*, Bristol: The Policy Press.

Bloom, B.S. (1964) *Stability and change in human characteristics*, New York: Wiley

Boddy, M. and Fudge, C. (eds) (1984) *Local socialism?*, London: Macmillan.

Bourdieu, P. (1986) 'The forms of capital', reprinted in Halsey, A.H., Lauder, H., Brown, P. and Wells, A.S. (eds) (1997) *Education, culture, economy and society*, Oxford: Oxford University Press.

Bradshaw, J. and Mayhew, E. (eds) (2005) *The well-being of children in the UK* (2nd edition), London: Save the Children.

Brooks-Gunn, J., Duncan, J.D. and Aber, J.L. (eds) (1997) *Neighborhood poverty. Volume I: context and consequences for children. Volume II: policy implications in studying neighborhoods*, New York: Russell Sage Foundation.

Campbell, B. (1984) *Wigan Pier revisited: poverty and politics in the 80s*, London: Virago Press.

Cannan, C. and Warren, C. (eds) (1997) *Social action with children and families: a community development approach to child and family welfare*, London: Routledge.

Central Advisory Council for Education (England) (CACE) (1967) *Children and their primary schools*, London: HMSO.

Coates, K. and Silburn, R. (1970) *Poverty: the forgotten Englishmen*, Harmondsworth: Penguin Books.

Coleman, J. (1988) 'Social capital in the creation of human capital', reprinted in Halsey, A.H., Lauder, H., Brown, P. and Wells, A.S. (eds) (1997) *Education, culture, economy and society*, Oxford: Oxford University Press.

Coulthard, M., Walker, A. and Morgan, A. (2002) *People's perceptions of their neighbourhood and community involvement. Results from the social capital module of the General Household Survey* 2000, London: Office for National Statistics, The Stationery Office.

Craig, G. with Adamson, S., Ali, N., Ali, S., Atkins, L., Dadze-Arthur, A., Elliott, C., McNamee, S. and Murtuja, B. (2007) *Sure Start and black and minority ethnic populations*, NESS/2007/FR/020, London: Department for Education and Skills.

Dench, G., Gavron, K. and Young, M. (2006) *The new East End: kinship, race and conflict*, London: Profile Books.

Dennis, N., Henriques, F. and Slaughter, C. (1956) *Coal is our life*, London: Eyre and Spottiswoode.

Department of the Environment, Transport and the Regions (DETR) (2000) *Measuring Multiple Deprivation at the Small Area Level: the Indices of Deprivation 2000*, London: Department of the Environment, Transport and the Regions.

Etzioni, A. (1997) *The new golden rule: community and morality in a democratic society*, London: Profile Books.

Frankenberg, R. (1966) *Communities in Britain: social life in town and country*, Harmondsworth: Penguin Books.

Frazer, E. (1999) *The problems of communitarian politics: unity and conflict*, Oxford: Oxford University Press.

Glass, N. (2006) 'Sure Start: where did it come from; where is it going?', *Journal of Children's Services*, 1(1), 51–7.

Hadley, R. and McGrath, M. (eds) (1980) *Going local: neighbourhood social services*, NCVO Occasional Paper 1, London: Bedford Square Press.

Hadley, R. and McGrath, M. (1984) *When social services are local: the Normanton experience*, London: Allen and Unwin.

Haezewindt, P. (2003) 'Investing in each other and the community: the role of social capital', *Social Trends*, 33: 19–26.

Halsey, A.H. (ed.) (1972) *Educational priority: volume 1: EPA problems and policies*, London: HMSO.

Hampton, W. (1970) *Democracy and community a study of politics in Sheffield*, London: Oxford University Press.

Harrington, M. (1962) *The other America: poverty in the United States*, Maryland: Penguin Books.

Harrison, P. (1983) *Inside the inner city – life under the cutting edge*, Harmondsworth: Penguin Books.

Henderson, P. (ed.) (1995) *Children and communities*, London: Pluto Press.

Hillery, G. (1963), 'Villages, cities and total institutions', *American Sociological Review*, 28: 779ff.

Hoggett, P. and Hambleton, R. (eds) (1987) *Decentralisation and democracy: localising public services*, Bristol: University of Bristol, School for Advanced Urban Studies.

Hunt, J. M. (1961), *Intelligence and experience*, New York: Ronald Press.

Hutchings, J., Bywater, T., Daley, D., Gardner, F., Jones, K., Eames, C. and Edwards, R.T. (2007) 'Pragmatic randomised controlled trial of a parenting intervention in Sure Start services for children at risk of developing conduct disorder', *British Medical Journal*, 334: 678.

Johnston, M. and Jowell, R. (2001) 'How robust is British civil society?', in Park, A., Curtice, J., Thomson, K., Jarvis, C. and Bromley, C. (eds) *British Social Attitudes: the 18th report: public policy, social ties*, National Centre for Social Research, London: Sage.

Killham, J. (1977) 'The idea of community in the English novel', *Nineteenth-Century Fiction*, 71(4): 379–96.

Knight, B. and Hayes, R. (1981) *Self help in the inner city*, London: London Voluntary Service Council.

Leonard, P. (ed.) (1975) *The sociology of community action*, Sociological Review Monograph 21, University of Keele.

Lewis, J. and Campbell, M. (2007) 'UK work/family balance policies and gender equality, 1997–2005', *Social Politics: International Studies in Gender, State & Society*, 14(1): 4–30.

Love, J.M., Kisker, E.E., Ross, C., Raikes, H., Constantine, J., Boller, K., Brooks-Gunn, J., Chazen-Coehn, R., Banks Tarvilo, L., Brady-Smith, C., Sidle Fulighi, A., Schochet, P.Z., Paulsell, D. and Vogel, C. (2005) 'The effectiveness of Early Head Start for 3-year-old children and their parents: lessons for policy and programs', *Developmental Psychology*, 41(6): 885–901.

Lupton, R. and Power, A. (2002) 'Social exclusion and neighbourhoods', in Hills, J., Le Grand, J. and Piachaud, D. (eds) *Understanding social exclusion*, Oxford: Oxford University Press.

Macdonald, K. and Grieco, M. (2007) 'Accessibility, mobility and connectivity: the changing frontiers of everyday routine', *Mobilities*, 2(1): 1–14.

Mayo, M. (1994) *Communities and caring: the mixed economy of welfare*, Basingstoke: Macmillan Press.

Midwinter, E. (1972) *Priority education: account of the Liverpool project*, Harmondsworth: Penguin.

Moorhouse, G. (1964) *The other England: Britain in the sixties*, Harmondsworth: Penguin.

Mumford, K. and Power, A. (2003) *East Enders: family and community in East London*, Bristol: Policy Press.

Nash, V. (ed.) (2002) *Reclaiming community*, London: IPPR.

Nash, V. with Christie, I. (2002) *Making sense of community*, London: IPPR.

National Evaluation of Sure Start (NESS) (2005a) *Early impacts of Sure Start Local Programmes on children and families: report of the Cross-sectional Study of 9 and 36 month old children and their families*, NESS/2005/FR/013, London: Department for Education and Skills.

National Evaluation of Sure Start (NESS) (2005b) *Variation in Sure Start Local Programmes' effectiveness: early preliminary findings: report of the NESS Programme Variability Study*, NESS/2005/FR/014, London: Department for Education and Skills.

Noble, M. and Smith, G. (1996) 'Two nations? Changing patterns of income and wealth in two contrasting areas', in Hills, J. (ed.) *New inequalities: the changing distribution of income and wealth in the United Kingdom*, Cambridge: Cambridge University Press.

Noble, M., Wright, G., Dibben, C., Smith, G., McLennan, D., Anttila, C. and Barnes, H. (2004) *The English Indices of Deprivation 2004*, London: Office of the Deputy Prime Minister, Neighbourhood Renewal Unit.

Parker, T. (1983) *The people of Providence: a housing estate and some of its inhabitants*, London: Hutchinson.

Payne, J. (1974) *Educational priority: volume 2: EPA surveys and statistics*, London: HMSO.

Putnam, R. (2000) *Bowling alone: the collapse and revival of American community*, New York: Simon and Schuster.

Putnam, R. (ed.) (2002) *Democracies in flux: the evolution of social capital in contemporary society*, New York: Oxford University Press.

Richardson, L. and Mumford, K. (2002) 'Community, neighbourhood and social infrastructure', in J. Hills, J. LeGrand and D. Piachavd (eds) *Understanding social exclusion*, Oxford: Oxford University Press.

Rose, N. (2000) 'Community, citizenship and the Third Way', *American Behavioral Scientist*, 43: 1395–411.

Royal Commission on Local Government (1969) *Community Attitudes Survey: England*, Research Study 9, London: HMSO.

Rutter, M. (2006) 'Is Sure Start an effective preventive intervention?', *Child and Adolescent Mental Health*, 11(3): 135–41.

Saegert, S., Thompson, J.P. and Warren, M.R. (eds) (2001) *Social capital and poor communities*, New York: Russell Sage Foundation.

Schuller, T., Baron, S. and Field, J. (2000) 'Social capital: a review and critique', in Baron, S., Field, J. and Schuller, T. (eds) *Social capital: critical perspectives*, Oxford: Oxford University Press.

Seabrook, J. (1984) *The idea of neighbourhood: what local politics should be about*, London: Pluto Press.

Seebohm Report (1968) *Report of the Committee on Local Authority and Allied Personal Social Services*, Cmnd.3703, London: HMSO.

Shankland, G., Willmott, P. and Jordan, D. (1977) *Inner London: policies for dispersal and balance: Final report of the Lambeth Inner Area Study*, London: HMSO.

Shonkoff, J.P. and Phillips, D. (2000) *From neurons to neighbourhoods: the science of early child development*, Washington D.C.: National Academy Press.

Sigala, M. and Smith, G. (2007) 'Neighbourhood dynamics and disadvantaged families with preschool children: the NNI Neighbourhood Tracking Study', in Smith, T., Smith, G., Coxon, K. and Sigala, M. *The Neighbourhood Nurseries Initiative National Evaluation Final Integrated Report*. SSU/2007/SF/024 and SSU/2007/FR/024, London: Department for Education and Skills.

Sisman, A. (2006) *The friendship: Wordsworth and Coleridge*, London: Harper Press.

Smith, G. (ed.) (1975) *Educational priority: volume 4: EPA the West Riding Project*, London: HMSO.

Smith, G., Smith, T. and Smith, T. (2007a) 'Whatever happened to EPAs? Part 2: Educational Priority Areas forty years on', *Forum*, 49(1): 141–56.

Smith, T. (1989) 'Decentralisation and community', *British Journal of Social Work*, 19: 137–48.

Smith, T. and Noble, M. (1995) *Education divides: poverty and schooling in the 1990s*, London: Child Poverty Action Group.

Smith, T., Smith, G., Coxon, K. and Sigala, M. (2007b) *The Neighbourhood Nurseries Initiative National Evaluation Final Integrated Report*, SSU/ 2007/ SF/ 024 and SSU/ 2007/ FR/ 024, London: Department for Education and Skills.

Smith, T., Coxon, K. and Sigala, M. (2007c) *The Neighbourhood Nurseries Initiative Implementation Study Final Report*, London: Department for Education and Skills.

Social Exclusion Unit (SEU) (1998) *Bringing Britain together: a national strategy for neighbourhood renewal*, Cm 4045, London: The Stationery Office.

Stacey, M. (1969) 'The myth of community studies', *British Journal of Sociology*, 20(2): 134–47.

Sylva, K., Melhuish, E., Sammons, P., Siraj-Blatchford, I. and Taggart, B. (2004) *The Effective Provision of Pre-School Education (EPPE) Project: Final Report: a longitudinal study funded by the DfES 1997–2004*, London: Department for Education and Skills.

Taylor, M. (1995) *Unleashing the potential: bringing residents to the centre of regeneration*, York: Joseph Rowntree Foundation.

Thatcher, M. (1987) *Woman's Own*, 31 October.

Townsend, P. (1957) *The family life of old people: an inquiry in East London*, London: Routledge and Kegan Paul.

Townsend, P. and Wedderburn, D. (1965) *The aged in the welfare state*, London: Bell

Williams, R. (1976) *Keywords: a vocabulary of culture and society*, London: Fontana.

Willmott, P. (1986) *Social networks, informal care and public policy*, London: Policy Studies Institute.

Willmott, P. and Young, M. (1960) *Family and class in a London suburb*, London: Routledge and Kegan Paul.

Work and Pensions Select Committee (2003) *Childcare for Working Parents*, HC564-I, Fifth Report, Session 2002–2003, London: The Stationery Office.

Young, M. and Willmott, P. (1957) *Family and kinship in East London*, London: Routledge and Kegan Paul.

Index

sociology and links to history 29
Soulside 34
South London Press 60
South Wales mining community 45–7
Spencer, R. 37
spirit of community 184
Stacey, J. 6, 12, 17, 18, 82
Stacey, Margaret 12, 13, 15, 16, 181–2, 198n
Stanley, L. 6, 80, 81, 82
Stein, Maurice 17
step-families 13–14
stories 29, 30, 38; sexual 52–3
Street Corner Society 31
Strode, M. 165
structural functionalism 4, 116, 117, 135
Sure Start 83, 182, 183, 191, 194, 195, 196, 197
Swann, M. 61
Swansea re-study 7, 114–28; baseline study 7, 16, 114–16; findings 119–30; methodological challenges 116–18; methods used 118–19
Sylva, K. 191
Szreter, S. 45, 87

Taylor, M. 191
technology 14, 88
telephones 141
Thane, P. 98
Thatcher, Margaret 182
theories of social change: cognitive dissonance 35; contemporary 16–19, 81–2, 116–17; data-free 129; modernisatation 135; structural functionalism 4, 116, 117, 135; transformation 80
Thompson, F. 15
Thompson, P. 3, 78, 79, 96
Thompson, R. 103
time, conceptions of 18–19, 81
'Timescapes' study 3
Tomlinson, S. 65–9
Tonnies, F. 12, 62
totemism 26
Townsend, Peter 134, 135, 140, 184, 187, 198n
Toynbee, P. 42
Tradition and Change 12
transgendered people 49
transnational families 62

trust 193, 194
Twin Rivers study 20

underclass 67, 73
unemployment 46, 155–8

values 12, 13, 14, 70, 81, 116; of the Caribbean community 72–3
Vencat, E.F. 36
venereal disease 104
Victor, C, 134
Village on the Border, A 29, 32
Vine, Samuel 104
violence 60, 72, 74
virtual communities 5, 14, 36–7, 38, 181, 185
Vuorela, U. 62

Wadsworth, M. 1
Waite, L. 164
Ward, R. 71
Warde, A. 80, 81
Warren, C. 182
Wedderburn, D. 198n
Weeks, J. 4, 6, 41, 42, 43, 50, 51, 52, 54, 62, 82
welfare state 1, 13, 134, 190
Wellman, B. 37, 137, 140
Wenger, G.C. 137, 138
Werbner, P. 35
When Prophecy Fails 35
Whyte, W.F. 31
Williams, Bill 11, 168
Williams, F. 81
Williams, Raymond 181
Willmott, Peter 13, 17, 29, 81, 85, 114, 134, 135, 140, 141, 142, 184, 185, 187, 188, 189
Willson, M. 37
Wilson, E. 135
Winter, I. 15
Wolfenden Report (1957) 43
Wolverhampton studies 134, 136, 138, 139, 141
women: as carers 106, 108, 110–11; continuity in the lives of 19; 'de-domestication' of 115; in the labour force 1, 17, 88, 126, 127–8, 129; maintaining kinship ties 115, 120, 124; mothers and daughters 124, 126, 128, 139, 185; sexuality of 45, 48